Multiple Choice Questions
in Hematology

Multiple Choice Questions in Hematology

Amin A. Alamin
MBBS, MD
Consultant &Associate Professor in Hematopathology, College of
Medicine, Taif University, Taif, Kingdom of Saudi Arabia

Content

Preface

This book has been written to serve as a comprehensive resource for medical students, residents, and practitioners who want to test their knowledge, improve their clinical skills, and prepare for exams. The questions within these pages cover a wide range of topics, from anemias to coagulopathies and from hematological malignancies to transfusion medicine.

Each question has been thoughtfully prepared to challenge the reader, and the accompanying explanations add clarity and understanding. Multiple-choice questions are well adapted to the dynamic nature of hematology, allowing for self-assessment and targeted learning.

As the field of hematology evolves with new discoveries and treatments, it is our hope that this book will be a useful resource in your journey of lifelong learning and professional development.

We wish you success as you explore the questions that lie ahead and may your pursuit of knowledge lead to improved outcomes for the patients in your care.

Amin A. Alamin, 2024

Dictation

"To my wife and daughters, the lights of my life."

Amin A. Alamin, 2024

Normal Ranges

This table displays the standard ranges for both the complete blood count (CBC) and coagulation test.

Tests	Units	Male	Female	Child
White blood cell count (WBC)	/mm3 (x10^3/µL)	4.5 - 11.0	4.5 - 11.0	5.0 - 17.0
Red blood cell count (RBC)	Millions/mm3 (x10^6/µL)	4.7 - 6.1	4.2 - 5.4	4.0 - 5.5
Hemoglobin (Hgb)	grams/dL	13.5 - 17.5	12.0 - 15.5	11.0 - 13.0
Hematocrit (Hct)	Percentage (%)	39 - 52	36 - 46	32 – 40
Mean corpuscular volume (MCV)	Fl (fL)	80 - 100	80 - 100	75 – 95
Mean corpuscular hemoglobin (MCH)	Picograms (pg)	27 - 34	27 - 34	26 – 33
Mean corpuscular hemoglobin concentration (MCHC)	Grams per deciliter (g/dL)	32 - 36	32 - 36	32 – 36
Red cell distribution width (RDW)	Percentage (%)	11.5 - 14.5	11.5 - 14.5	11.5 - 14.5
Platelet count	Thousands/mm3 (x10^3/µL)	150 - 450	150 - 450	150 – 450
Neutrophils (absolute value)	Thousands/mm3 (x10^3/µL)	1.8 - 7.7	1.8 - 7.7	1.5 - 8.5
Lymphocytes (absolute value)	Thousands/mm3 (x10^3/µL)	1.0 - 4.8	1.0 - 4.8	1.5 - 8.5
Monocytes (absolute value)	Thousands/mm3 (x10^3/µL)	0.2 - 1.1	0.2 - 1.1	0.2 - 1.1
Eosinophils (absolute value)	Thousands/mm3 (x10^3/µL)	0.0 - 0.5	0.0 - 0.5	0.0 - 0.5
Basophils (absolute value)	Thousands/mm3 (x10^3/µL)	0.0 - 0.3	0.0 - 0.3	0.0 - 0.3
Prothrombin time (PT)	Seconds (sec)	11.0 - 13.5	11.0 - 13.5	11.0 - 13.5
International normalized ratio (INR)	Ratio (-)	0.85 - 1.15	0.85 - 1.15	0.85 - 1.15
Activated partial thromboplastin time (aPTT)	Seconds (sec)	24.0 - 36.0	24.0 - 36.0	24.0 - 36.0

Abbreviations

AA	Aplastic Anemia
ABO	Blood group system
ACD	Anemia of Chronic Disease
ADAMTS13	A disintegrin And Metalloproteinase with a thrombospondin type 1 motif, member 13
ALL	Acute Lymphoblastic Leukemia
AML	Acute Myeloid Leukemia
APL	Acute Promyelocytic Leukemia
APS	Antiphospholipid Syndrome
ATRA	All-Trans Retinoic Acid
B12	Vitamin B12
BCL2	B-Cell Lymphoma 2
BCL6	B-Cell Lymphoma 6
BCR: ABL1	Is a fusion gene linked to chronic myeloid leukemia and acute lymphoblastic leukemia
CCND1	Cyclin D1
CD	Cluster of Differentiation
CLL	Chronic Lymphocytic Leukemia
CLL/SLL	Chronic Lymphocytic Leukemia/Small Lymphocytic Lymphoma
CML	Chronic Myeloid Leukemia
COX	Cyclooxygenase
DDAVP	Desmopressin
D-dimer -	A fibrin degradation product used to assess the presence of blood clots.
DIC	Disseminated Intravascular Coagulation
DLBCL	Diffuse Large B-Cell Lymphoma
DNA	Deoxyribonucleic Acid
DVT	Deep Vein Thrombosis
eGFR	Estimated Glomerular Filtration Rate
FIP1L1-PDGFRA	Fusion of FIP1-like-1 with platelet-derived growth factor receptor alpha
FL	Follicular Lymphoma
G6PD	Glucose-6-Phosphate Dehydrogenase
GIST	Gastrointestinal Stromal Tumor
GPT	Glutamate Pyruvate Transaminase (Enzyme)
HIT	Heparin-Induced Thrombocytopenia
HIV	Human Immunodeficiency Virus
HS	Hereditary Spherocytosis
IDA	Iron Deficiency Anemia
Ig	Immunoglobulin
IgA	Immunoglobulin A
IgE	Immunoglobulin E

IgG	Immunoglobulin G
IgM	Immunoglobulin M
IL-1	Interleukin-1
IL-6	Interleukin-6
ITP	Immune Thrombocytopenic Purpura
JAK2	Janus kinase 2
LDH	Lactate Dehydrogenase
LGLL	Large Granular Lymphocytic Leukemia
MDS	Myelodysplastic Syndrome
MGUS	Monoclonal gammopathy of undetermined significance
TdT	Terminal deoxynucleotidyl transferase
MPO	Myeloperoxidase
MYC	Myelocytomatosis Oncogene
MYD88	Myeloid Differentiation Primary Response 88
NF-κB	Nuclear Factor Kappa B
NSAIDs	Nonsteroidal Anti-Inflammatory Drugs
PCR	Polymerase Chain Reaction
Ph	Philadelphia Chromosome
PLL	Prolymphocytic Leukemia
Rh	Rhesus factor
SF3B1	Splicing Factor 3B Subunit 1
SS	Sezary Syndrome
TACO	Transfusion-Associated Circulatory Overload
TIBC	Total Iron-Binding Capacity
TKI	Tyrosine Kinase Inhibitor
TNF-alpha	Tumor Necrosis Factor-alpha
TP53	Tumor Protein p53
TRALI	Transfusion-Related Acute Lung Injury
TTP	Thrombotic Thrombocytopenic Purpura

Section 1:

Single Best Answers Questions 1-125

This section comprises 100 single best answer questions covering a wide range of hematological disorders. Designed for both beginners and experts, these questions aim to assess and strengthen your understanding of basic concepts. Each question is followed by multiple-choice options, with only one being the most accurate. Use this resource not just for assessment but also to deepen your insight into clinical reasoning and evidence-based practices in hematology.

Answers and explanation will be found on pages 76-87.

SBA 1.
What is the primary site of erythropoiesis in adults?
a) Liver
b) Spleen
c) Bone marrow
d) Lymph nodes
e) Kidneys

SBA 2
Which hormone regulates erythropoiesis?
a) Testosterone
b) Erythropoietin
c) Growth hormone
d) Thyroxine
e) Insulin

SBA 3
What triggers the release of erythropoietin?
a) High oxygen levels
b) Low oxygen levels
c) High carbon dioxide levels
d) Nutrient abundance
e) Inflammation

SBA 4
Which vitamin is essential for DNA synthesis during erythropoiesis?
a) Vitamin A
b) Vitamin B6
c) Vitamin B12
d) Vitamin C
e) Vitamin D

SBA 5
What is the first recognizable precursor in the erythroid lineage?
a) Myeloblast
b) Lymphoblast
c) Proerythroblast
d) Megakaryoblast
e) Monoblast

SBA 6
Which mineral is required for hemoglobin synthesis in erythropoiesis?
a) Calcium
b) Iron
c) Magnesium
d) Potassium
e) Zinc

SBA 7
What is the effect of erythropoietin on bone marrow?
a) It decreases red blood cell production.
b) It increases white blood cell production.
c) It increases red blood cell production.
e) It has no effect on bone marrow.
SBA 8
Which of the following cells is the last nucleated stage in erythropoiesis?
a) Reticulocyte
b) Normoblast
c) Myelocyte
d) Orthochromatophilic erythroblast
e) Polychromatophilic erythroblast
SBA 9
During erythropoiesis, the reduction in cell size is accompanied by
a) Increase in cytoplasmic volume.
b) Decrease in cytoplasmic volume.
c) Increase in nuclear size.
d) Decrease in hemoglobin content.
e) Increase in cell number.
SBA 10
What is the fate of erythroblasts that fail to synthesize sufficient hemoglobin during erythropoiesis?
a) They become white blood cells.
b) They are stored in the spleen.
c) They undergo apoptosis.
d) They circulate as immature red blood cells.
e) They differentiate into platelets.
SBA 11
Which of the following is a common cause of anemia in the elderly?
a) Hemoglobinopathies
b) Chronic blood loss
c) Sideroblastic anemia
d) Pure red cell aplasia
e) Paroxysmal nocturnal hemoglobinuria
SBA 12
What is the most likely diagnosis in a patient with anemia, jaundice, and an elevated reticulocyte count?
a) Iron deficiency anemia
b) Pernicious anemia
c) Aplastic anemia
d) Hemolytic anemia
e) Anemia of chronic disease

SBA 13
Which of the following laboratory findings is indicative of iron deficiency anemia?
a) Increased mean corpuscular volume (MCV)
b) Decreased serum ferritin
c) Increased serum iron
d) Decreased total iron-binding capacity (TIBC)
e) Increased serum transferrin

SBA 14
What is the most common type of anemia worldwide?
a) Sickle cell anemia
b) Pernicious anemia
c) Aplastic anemia
d) Iron deficiency anemia

SBA 15
Which vitamin deficiency can lead to megaloblastic anemia?
a) Vitamin A
b) Vitamin C
c) Vitamin B12
d) Vitamin D
e) Vitamin E

SBA 16
What is the characteristic shape of red blood cells in sickle cell anemia?
a) Spherocytes
b) Elliptocytes
c) Schistocytes
d) Sickle cells
e) Stomatocytes

SBA 17
Which of the following is not a cause of hemolytic anemia?
a) Autoimmune disorders
b) Genetic defects
c) Infectious agents d
) Chronic kidney disease
e) Medications

SBA 18
What is the main treatment for thalassemia major?
a) Oral iron supplements
b) Regular blood transfusions
c) High doses of vitamin B12
d) Splenectomy
e) Bone marrow transplant

SBA 19

Which of the following is a characteristic finding in iron deficiency anemia?

a) High serum ferritin

b) Low total iron-binding capacity (TIBC)

c) High mean corpuscular volume (MCV)

d) Low serum iron

e) High reticulocyte count

SBA 20

What is the primary cause of anemia of chronic disease?

a) Nutritional deficiencies

b) Bone marrow failure

c) Chronic inflammation

d) Hemolysis

e) Blood loss

SBA 21

Which of the following is not typically associated with pernicious anemia?

a) Vitamin B12 deficiency

b) Autoimmune gastritis

c) Neurological symptoms

d) Elevated mean corpuscular volume (MCV)

e) Elevated serum iron

SBA 22

What is the inheritance pattern of hereditary spherocytosis?

a) X-linked recessive

b) Autosomal dominant

c) Autosomal recessive

d) Mitochondrial

e) Multifactorial

SBA 23

Which of the following is a common symptom of anemia?

a) Jaundice

b) Hypertension

c) Fatigue

d) Weight gain

e) Hyperactivity

SBA 24

Aplastic anemia is characterized by

a) Overproduction of red blood cells

b) Deficiency of intrinsic factor

c) Bone marrow failure

d) High levels of hemoglobin

e) Iron overload

SBA 25
Which laboratory finding is typical for hemolytic anemia?
a) Low reticulocyte count
b) Low lactate dehydrogenase (LDH)
c) High haptoglobin
d) Elevated indirect bilirubin
e) Normal urine hemosiderin

SBA 26
What is the effect of lead poisoning on erythropoiesis?
a) It stimulates erythropoiesis.
b) It has no effect on erythropoiesis.
c) It inhibits erythropoiesis.
d) It increases iron absorption.
e) It increases erythrocyte lifespan.

SBA 27
Which of the following is a cause of macrocytic anemia?
a) Iron deficiency
b) Vitamin B12 deficiency
c) Thalassemia
d) Lead poisoning
e) G6PD deficiency

SBA 28
What is the most common cause of anemia in pregnancy?
a) Folic acid deficiency
b) Iron deficiency
c) Vitamin B12 deficiency
d) Hemolysis
e) Chronic disease

SBA 29
Which of the following is not a typical feature of Fanconi anemia?
a) Bone marrow failure
b) Increased risk of malignancies
c) Macrocytosis
d) High reticulocyte count
e) Congenital abnormalities

SBA 30
What is the Coombs test used for?
a) Detecting iron deficiency
b) Measuring hemoglobin levels
c) Diagnosing thalassemia
d) Detecting antibodies against red blood cells
e) Assessing bone marrow function

SBA 31

Which of the following is a cause of normocytic anemia?

a) Chronic liver disease

b) Chronic renal failure

c) Vitamin C deficiency

d) Copper deficiency

e) Zinc deficiency

SBA 32

Which of the following is not a characteristic of infectious mononucleosis?

a) Fever

b) Pharyngitis

c) Splenomegaly

d) Thrombocytopenia

e) Atypical lymphocytes

SBA 33

What is the most common cause of neutrophilia?

a) Viral infections

b) Bacterial infections

c) Allergic reactions

d) Parasitic infections

e) Medications

SBA 34

Which leukocyte disorder is characterized by an absolute increase in the number of eosinophils?

a) Eosinophilia

b) Basophilia

c) Lymphocytosis

d) Monocytosis

e) Neutropenia

SBA 35

Leukocytosis can be a physiological response to

a) Sleep

b) Exercise

c) Eating

d) All of the above

e) None of the above

SBA 36

Which of the following is a benign disorder characterized by the presence of large granular lymphocytes?

a) Acute lymphoblastic leukemia

b) Chronic lymphocytic leukemia

c) Large granular lymphocytic leukemia

d) Hairy cell leukemia

e) T-cell acute lymphoblastic leukemia

SBA 37

Pelger-Huët anomaly is associated with
a) Hypersegmented neutrophils
b) Hyposegmented neutrophils
c) Giant platelets
d) Atypical lymphocytes
e) Eosinopenia

SBA 38

Which condition is characterized by an increased number of circulating monocytes?
a) Monocytopenia
b) Monocytosis
c) Lymphopenia
d) Eosinopenia
e) Basopenia

SBA 39

What is the typical cause of lymphocytosis in children?
a) Bacterial infections
b) Viral infections
c) Allergic reactions
d) Autoimmune diseases
e) Medications

SBA 40

Which of the following is not a typical feature of chronic lymphocytic leukemia (CLL)?
a) Lymphadenopathy
b) Splenomegaly
c) Increased risk of infections
d) High neutrophil count
e) Presence of smudge cells

SBA 41

Reactive lymphocytosis can occur due to
a) Smoking
b) Stress
c) Exercise
d) All of the above
e) None of the above

SBA 42

Which of the following is not a function of platelets?
a) Hemostasis
b) Blood clot retraction
c) Phagocytosis
d) Release of growth factors
e) Adhesion to damaged endothelium

SBA 43

What is the most common inherited bleeding disorder?

a) Hemophilia A

b) Hemophilia B

c) Von Willebrand disease

d) Factor XI deficiency

e) Glanzmann thrombasthenia

SBA 44

Which coagulation factor is deficient in Hemophilia A?

a) Factor VIII

b) Factor IX

c) Factor XI

d) Factor V

e) Factor X

SBA 45

What is the primary initial treatment for acute Immune Thrombocytopenic Purpura (ITP)?

a) Platelet transfusion

b) Intravenous immunoglobulin (IVIG)

c) Corticosteroids

d) Splenectomy

e) Antifibrinolytic agents

SBA 46

Which laboratory test is prolonged in Hemophilia A?

a) Prothrombin time (PT)

b) Thrombin time (TT)

c) Activated partial thromboplastin time (aPTT)

d) Bleeding time (BT)

e) Platelet count

SBA 47

Disseminated Intravascular Coagulation (DIC) is characterized by

a) Increased platelet count

b) Prolonged PT and aPTT

c) Normal fibrinogen levels

d) Decreased D-dimer

e) Isolated thrombocytopenia

SBA 48

Which of the following is a cause of acquired thrombocytopenia?

a) May-Hegglin anomaly

b) Bernard-Soulier syndrome

c) Drug-induced thrombocytopenia

d) Glanzmann thrombasthenia

e) Chédiak-Higashi syndrome

SBA 49
Von Willebrand disease primarily affects
a) Platelet aggregation
b) Fibrinolysis
c) Secondary hemostasis
d) Primary hemostasis
e) Red blood cell morphology

SBA 50
What is the treatment of choice for patients with Hemophilia A and inhibitors to Factor VIII?
a) Desmopressin (DDAVP)
b) Recombinant Factor VIII
c) Bypassing agents like recombinant Factor VIIa
d) Fresh frozen plasma (FFP)
e) Cryoprecipitate

SBA 51
Which of the following is not typically associated with thrombotic thrombocytopenic purpura (TTP)?
a) Fever
b) Microangiopathic hemolytic anemia
c) Neurological symptoms
d) Renal impairment
e) Elevated prothrombin time (PT)

SBA 52
What is the most common cause of acquired coagulation factor deficiency?
a) Hemophilia A
b) Vitamin K deficiency
c) Liver disease
d) Von Willebrand disease
e) Antiphospholipid syndrome

SBA 53
Which of the following is a characteristic finding in Glanzmann thrombasthenia?
a) Deficiency of GPIIb/IIIa receptors on platelets
b) Deficiency of von Willebrand factor
c) Deficiency of Factor VIII
d) Presence of antiplatelet antibodies
e) Elevated D-dimer levels

SBA 54
Which factor is involved in both the intrinsic and extrinsic pathways of the coagulation cascade?
a) Factor VII
b) Factor VIII
c) Factor IX

d) Factor X
e) Factor V
SBA 55
What is the mainstay of treatment for von Willebrand disease**?**
a) Vitamin K supplementation
b) Desmopressin (DDAVP)
c) Platelet transfusion
d) Recombinant Factor VIII
e) Antifibrinolytic agents
SBA 56
Which of the following is a common cause of acquired Vitamin K deficiency?
a) Prolonged antibiotic therapy
b) Excessive intake of green leafy vegetables
c) Genetic mutation in the VKORC1 gene
d) Overproduction of bile acids
e) High doses of vitamin E supplementation
SBA 57
In patients with liver disease, which coagulation factor is typically not decreased?
a) Factor V
b) Factor VII
c) Factor VIII
d) Factor IX
e) Factor X
SBA 58
What is the primary mechanism of action of heparin?
a) Inhibition of thrombin
b) Activation of antithrombin III
c) Direct inhibition of Factor Xa
d) Inhibition of platelet aggregation
e) Activation of protein C
SBA 59
Which of the following is not a typical feature of Hemophilia B?
a) X-linked recessive inheritance
b) Deficiency of Factor IX
c) Prolonged bleeding time
d) Normal platelet count
e) Prolonged aPTT
SBA 60
Which of the following is a direct oral anticoagulant (DOAC) that inhibits Factor Xa?
a) Warfarin
b) Heparin
c) Dabigatran

d) Rivaroxaban
e) Argatroban

SBA 61

A patient with a platelet count of 20,000/µL is at risk for:

a) Thrombosis
b) Hemarthrosis
c) Spontaneous bleeding
d) Vitamin K deficiency
e) Disseminated intravascular coagulation

SBA 62

What is the primary treatment for heparin-induced thrombocytopenia (HIT)?

a) Continue heparin and monitor platelet count
b) Discontinue heparin and start warfarin
c) Discontinue heparin and start a non-heparin anticoagulant
d) Platelet transfusion
e) Intravenous immunoglobulin (IVIG)

SBA 63

Which of the following is not a common side effect of anticoagulant therapy?

a) Bleeding
b) Bruising
c) Thrombocytopenia
d) Hypertension
e) Hematuria

SBA 64

The presence of schistocytes on a peripheral blood smear is indicative of

a) Iron deficiency anemia
b) Vitamin B12 deficiency
c) Microangiopathic hemolytic anemia
d) Sickle cell anemia
e) G6PD deficiency

SBA 65

Which of the following is a characteristic finding in essential thrombocythemia?

a) Low platelet count
b) High platelet count
c) Prolonged bleeding time
d) Decreased megakaryocytes in the bone marrow
e) Normal coagulation test results

SBA 66

What is the most common cause of thrombocytopenia in hospitalized patients?

a) Bone marrow failure
b) Immune thrombocytopenic purpura (ITP)

c) Drug-induced thrombocytopenia
d) Sepsis
e) Hemolytic uremic syndrome (HUS)

SBA 67

Which of the following tests measures the intrinsic pathway of the coagulation cascade?
a) Prothrombin time (PT)
b) Thrombin time (TT)
c) Activated partial thromboplastin time (aPTT)
d) Platelet function assay
e) Bleeding time

SBA 68

What is the treatment of choice for patients with severe thrombotic thrombocytopenic purpura (TTP)?
a) Corticosteroids
b) Platelet transfusion
c) Plasma exchange
d) Intravenous immunoglobulin (IVIG)
e) Splenectomy

SBA 69

Which of the following conditions is associated with a prolonged prothrombin time (PT)?
a) Hemophilia A
b) Von Willebrand disease
c) Vitamin K deficiency
d) Glanzmann thrombasthenia
e) Bernard-Soulier syndrome

SBA 70

What is the most common cause of inherited thrombophilia?
a) Protein C deficiency
b) Protein S deficiency
c) Antithrombin deficiency
d) Factor V Leiden mutation
e) Prothrombin G20210A mutation

SBA 71

Which of the following is not typically associated with antiphospholipid syndrome (APS)?
a) Recurrent miscarriages
b) Venous thromboembolism
c) Arterial thrombosis
d) Thrombocytopenia
e) Elevated white blood cell count

SBA 72

What is the primary function of von Willebrand factor (vWF)?

a) To carry oxygen to tissues

b) To mediate platelet adhesion to subendothelial collagen

c) To activate the extrinsic pathway of coagulation

d) To serve as a cofactor for Factor VIII

e) To lyse blood clots

SBA 73

Which of the following is a common complication of deep vein thrombosis (DVT)?

a) Hemophilia

b) Pulmonary embolism

c) Hemarthrosis

d) Hemolytic anemia

e) Disseminated intravascular coagulation

SBA 74

What is the primary treatment for essential thrombocythemia?

a) Hydroxyurea

b) Aspirin

c) Anagrelide

d) All of the above

e) None of the above

SBA 75

Which of the following is not a typical feature of disseminated intravascular coagulation (DIC)?

a) Increased fibrin degradation products

b) Thrombocytopenia

c) Prolonged bleeding time

d) Normal D-dimer levels

e) Schistocytes on peripheral blood smear

SBA 76

Which hematological malignancy is characterized by the Philadelphia chromosome?

a) Acute lymphoblastic leukemia (ALL)

b) Chronic myeloid leukemia (CML)

c) Multiple myeloma

d) Hodgkin lymphoma

e) Non-Hodgkin lymphoma

SBA 77

What is the most common type of non-Hodgkin lymphoma?

a) Burkitt lymphoma

b) Follicular lymphoma

c) Mantle cell lymphoma

d) Diffuse large B-cell lymphoma

e) Lymphoblastic lymphoma

SBA 78

Which of the following is a hallmark feature of multiple myeloma?

a) Reed-Sternberg cells

b) Auer rods

c) Bence Jones proteins

d) Smudge cells

e) Pelger-Huët anomaly

SBA 79

What is the primary treatment for acute promyelocytic leukemia (APL)?

a) Chemotherapy with anthracyclines

b) All-trans retinoic acid (ATRA)

c) High-dose corticosteroids

d) Stem cell transplantation

e) Radiation therapy

SBA 80

Which of the following is not a B-cell marker?

a) CD19

b) CD20

c) CD3

d) CD22

e) CD79a

SBA 81

What is the most common presenting symptom of Hodgkin lymphoma?

a) Bone pain

b) Night sweats

c) Painless lymphadenopathy

d) Weight loss

e) Fever

SBA 82

Which genetic mutation is commonly associated with chronic lymphocytic leukemia (CLL)?

a) JAK2 V617F

b) BCR-ABL1

c) TP53

d) FLT3-ITD

e) NPM1

SBA 83

What is the characteristic cell found in Hodgkin lymphoma?

a) Lymphoblast

b) Myeloblast

c) Reed-Sternberg cell

d) Plasma cell

e) Hairy cell

SBA 84
Which of the following is a risk factor for developing acute myeloid leukemia (AML)?
a) Smoking
b) Previous chemotherapy or radiation therapy
c) Genetic syndromes like Down syndrome
d) All of the above
e) None of the above

SBA 85
What is the most common cytogenetic abnormality in adult acute lymphoblastic leukemia (ALL)?
a) t(9;22)(q34;q11.2)
b) t(15;17)(q22;q12)
c) t(8;21)(q22;q22)
d) t(12;21)(p13;q22)
e) t(14;18)(q32;q21)

SBA 86
Which of the following is a common complication of myelodysplastic syndromes (MDS)?
a) Transformation to acute leukemia
b) Solid tumors
c) Lymphoma
d) Benign tumors
e) None of the above

SBA 87
What is the primary function of the CD20 molecule found on B cells?
a) Signal transduction
b) Phagocytosis
c) Antigen presentation
d) Cell adhesion
e) Cytokine production

SBA 88
Which of the following is not a typical symptom of chronic myeloid leukemia (CML)?
a) Fatigue
b) Splenomegaly
c) Easy bruising
d) Hypercalcemia
e) Night sweats

SBA 89
What is the most common presenting symptom of multiple myeloma?
a) Lymphadenopathy
b) Bone pain
c) Hepatomegaly

d) Skin rash

e) Hemoptysis

SBA 90

Which of the following is a characteristic finding in Waldenström macroglobulinemia?

a) Hyperviscosity syndrome

b) Hypercalcemia

c) Philadelphia chromosome

d) Auer rods

e) Reed-Sternberg cells

SBA 91

Which of the following is a common treatment for follicular lymphoma?

a) All-trans retinoic acid (ATRA)

b) Imatinib

c) Rituximab

d) Thalidomide

e) Hydroxyurea

SBA 92

What is the most common type of leukemia in children?

a) Acute myeloid leukemia (AML)

b) Chronic lymphocytic leukemia (CLL)

c) Acute lymphoblastic leukemia (ALL)

d) Chronic myeloid leukemia (CML)

e) Hairy cell leukemia

SBA 93

Which of the following is a poor prognostic indicator in AML?

a) t(8;21)(q22;q22)

b) t(15;17)(q22;q12)

c) Complex karyotype

d) NPM1 mutation without FLT3-ITD

e) CEBPA biallelic mutation

SBA 94

Which of the following is not a common side effect of chemotherapy for hematological malignancies?

a) Nausea and vomiting

b) Hair loss

c) Neuropathy

d) Hypertension

e) Myelosuppression

SBA 95

Which of the following is a characteristic feature of Burkitt lymphoma?

a) Presence of Philadelphia chromosome

b) Translocation t(14;18)(q32;q21)

c) Translocation t(8;14)(q24;q32)

d) Hyperdiploidy

e) JAK2 V617F mutation

SBA 96

What is the primary cause of primary polycythemia (polycythemia vera)?

a) Dehydration

b) Chronic hypoxia

c) Renal disease

d) Mutation in the JAK2 gene

e) High altitude

SBA 97

Which of the following symptoms is not commonly associated with polycythemia vera?

a) Headaches

b) Dizziness

c) Hypertension

d) Tachycardia

e) Pruritus after a hot shower

SBA 98

What is the most common complication of secondary polycythemia?

a) Thrombosis

b) Leukemia

c) Heart failure

d) Infection

e) Bleeding

SBA 99

Which of the following is a diagnostic criterion for polycythemia vera?

a) Elevated white blood cell count

b) Low erythropoietin levels

c) Presence of the Philadelphia chromosome

d) Elevated red blood cell mass

e) Decreased platelet count

SBA 100

What is the initial treatment of choice for reducing hematocrit in polycythemia vera?

a) Chemotherapy

b) Phlebotomy

c) Aspirin

d) Hydroxyurea

e) Interferon-alpha

SBA 101

Which of the following is not typically associated with thrombocytopenia in multiple myeloma?

a) Bone marrow infiltration by plasma cells

b) Increased platelet destruction

c) Nutritional deficiencies
d) Myelosuppressive chemotherapy
e) Direct platelet production by myeloma cells

SBA 102

What is the primary mechanism leading to anemia in patients with multiple myeloma?

a) Hemolysis
b) Blood loss
c) Bone marrow replacement by malignant plasma cells
d) Vitamin B12 deficiency
e) Autoimmune destruction

SBA 103

Which of the following is a characteristic finding on the peripheral blood smear of a patient with multiple myeloma?

a) Spherocytes
b) Schistocytes
c) Rouleaux formation
d) Target cells
e) Howell-Jolly bodies

SBA 104

In multiple myeloma, the presence of which of the following is a poor prognostic marker?

a) Elevated serum albumin
b) Low serum beta-2 microglobulin
c) High serum calcium
d) Low serum lactate dehydrogenase (LDH)
e) Elevated serum creatinine

SBA 105

Which of the following is not a common clinical feature of multiple myeloma?

a) Bone pain
b) Recurrent infections
c) Weight loss
d) Thrombocytosis
e) Anemia

SBA 106

What is the most common blood type in the world?

a) A+
b) B+
c) AB+
e) O+
e) O-

SBA 107
What is the universal donor blood type?
a) A+
b) B+
c) AB+
d) O+
e) O-
SBA 108
What is the universal recipient blood type?
a) A+
b) B+
c) AB+
d) O+
e) O-
SBA 109
What is the Rh factor and how does it affect blood transfusion?
a) It is a protein on the surface of the red blood cells that determines the blood type
b) It is a gene that codes for the production of antigens on the surface of the red blood cells
c) It is an antibody that is produced by the immune system in response to foreign antigens
d) It is a substance that is added to the blood to prevent clotting during transfusion
e) It is a hormone that regulates the blood pressure and volume
SBA 110
What is the most common complication of blood transfusion?
a) Hemolytic reaction
b) Allergic reaction
c) Febrile reaction
d) Transfusion-related acute lung injury (TRALI)
e) Transfusion-associated circulatory overload (TACO)
SBA 111
What is the most serious complication of blood transfusion?
a) Hemolytic reaction
b) Allergic reaction
c) Febrile reaction
d) Transfusion-related acute lung injury (TRALI)
e) Transfusion-associated circulatory overload (TACO)
SBA 112
What is the most common infectious risk of blood transfusion?
a) HIV
b) Hepatitis B
c) Hepatitis C

d) Syphilis
e) Malaria
SBA 113
What is the most rare infectious risk of blood transfusion?
a) HIV
b) Hepatitis B
c) Hepatitis C
d) Syphilis
e) Malaria
SBA 114
What is the recommended blood product for patients with severe anemia?
a) Whole blood
b) Packed red blood cells
c) Fresh frozen plasma
d) Platelets
e) Cryoprecipitate
SBA 115
What is the recommended blood product for patients with severe bleeding?
a) Whole blood
b) Packed red blood cells
c) Fresh frozen plasma
d) Platelets
e) Cryoprecipitate
SBA 116
What is the recommended blood product for patients with coagulation
disorders?
a) Whole blood
b) Packed red blood cells
c) Fresh frozen plasma
d) Platelets
e) Cryoprecipitate
SBA 117
What is the recommended blood product for patients with
thrombocytopenia?
a) Whole blood
b) Packed red blood cells
c) Fresh frozen plasma
d) Platelets
e) Cryoprecipitate
SBA 118
What is the recommended blood product for patients with hemophilia A?
a) Whole blood
b) Packed red blood cells
c) Fresh frozen plasma

d) Platelets

e) Cryoprecipitate

SBA 119

What is the recommended blood product for patients with sickle cell disease?

a) Whole blood

b) Packed red blood cells

c) Fresh frozen plasma

d) Platelets

e) Cryoprecipitate

SBA 120

What is the recommended blood product for patients with massive blood loss due to trauma or surgery?

a) Whole blood

b) Packed red blood cells

c) Fresh frozen plasma

d) Platelets

e) Cryoprecipitate

SBA 121

What is the recommended blood product for patients with thrombotic thrombocytopenic purpura (TTP)?

a) Whole blood

b) Packed red blood cells

c) Fresh frozen plasma

d) Platelets

e) Cryoprecipitate

SBA 122

What is the recommended blood product for patients with disseminated intravascular coagulation (DIC)?

a) Whole blood

b) Packed red blood cells

c) Fresh frozen plasma

d) Platelets

e) Cryoprecipitate

SBA 123

What is the recommended blood product for patients with acute leukemia?

a) Whole blood

b) Packed red blood cells

c) Fresh frozen plasma

d) Platelets

e) Cryoprecipitate

SBA 124
What is the recommended blood product for patients with iron deficiency anemia?
a) Whole blood
b) Packed red blood cells
c) Fresh frozen plasma
d) Platelets
e) Cryoprecipitate
SBA 125
Which blood product is most suitable for treating newborn babies who have anemia due to their mother's antibodies attacking their red blood cells?
a) Whole blood
b) Packed red blood cells
c) Fresh frozen plasma
d) Platelets
e) Cryoprecipitate

Section 2
Scenario-based MCQ Questions 1-85

This section (questions 101–200) comprises scenario-based multiple-choice questions designed to reflect real-world clinical situations in hematology. Aimed at testing both theoretical knowledge and practical decision-making skills, these questions present diverse clinical vignettes, challenging you to integrate principles with evidence-based medicine. We believe that these scenario-based questions will help you comprehend the diverse nature of hematology and give you the confidence to succeed in academic and clinical settings.

Answers and explanations will be found on pages 91 – 112

SBQ 1.

A 65-year-old man presents to the clinic with fatigue, pallor, and dyspnea on exertion. His complete blood count shows a hemoglobin of 9.5 g/dL, a mean corpuscular volume (MCV) of 72 fL, and a red cell distribution width (RDW) of 18%. His serum iron level is low, his total iron-binding capacity (TIBC) is high, and his ferritin level is low. What is the most likely type of anemia in this patient?

a) Iron deficiency anemia

b) Anemia of chronic disease

c) Thalassemia

d) Sideroblastic anemia

e) Vitamin b12 deficiency anemia

SBQ 2

A 25-year-old woman presents to the clinic with fatigue, pallor, and jaundice. Her complete blood count shows a hemoglobin of 8.0 g/dL, a mean corpuscular volume (MCV) of 68 fL, and a red cell distribution width (RDW) of 15%. Her serum iron level is normal, her total iron-binding capacity (TIBC) is normal, and her ferritin level is normal. Her peripheral blood smear shows target cells and basophilic stippling. What is the most likely type of anemia in this patient?

a) Iron deficiency anemia

b) Anemia of chronic disease

c) Thalassemia

d) Sideroblastic anemia

e) Vitamin b12 deficiency anemia

SBQ 3

A 45-year-old man presents to the clinic with fatigue, pallor, and weight loss. He has a history of rheumatoid arthritis and chronic kidney disease. His complete blood count shows a hemoglobin of 10.0 g/dL, a mean corpuscular volume (MCV) of 84 fL, and a red cell distribution width (RDW) of 14%. His serum iron level is low, his total iron-binding capacity (TIBC) is low, and his ferritin level is high. What is the most likely type of anemia in this patient?

a) Iron deficiency anemia

b) Anemia of chronic disease

c) Thalassemia

d) Sideroblastic anemia

e) Vitamin b12 deficiency anemia

SBQ 4

A 35-year-old woman presents to the clinic with fatigue, pallor, and paresthesias. She has a history of pernicious anemia and gastric bypass surgery. Her complete blood count shows a hemoglobin of 9.0 g/dL, a mean corpuscular volume (MCV) of 110 fL, and a red cell distribution width (RDW) of 16%. Her serum vitamin B12 level is low and her serum folate level is

normal. Her peripheral blood smear shows macrocytic (large) and oval-shaped red blood cells and hypersegmented neutrophils. What is the most likely type of anemia in this patient?
a) Iron deficiency anemia
b) Anemia of chronic disease
c) Thalassemia
d) Sideroblastic anemia
e) Vitamin B12 deficiency anemia

SBQ 5

A 55-year-old man presents to the clinic with fatigue, pallor, and abdominal pain. He has a history of alcohol abuse and chronic pancreatitis. His complete blood count shows a hemoglobin of 10.5 g/dL, a mean corpuscular volume (MCV) of 96 fL, and a red cell distribution width (RDW) of 15%. His serum iron level is high, his total iron-binding capacity (TIBC) is low, and his ferritin level is high. His bone marrow biopsy shows ringed sideroblasts. What is the most likely type of anemia in this patient?
a) Iron deficiency anemia
b) Anemia of chronic disease
c) Thalassemia
d) Sideroblastic anemia
e) Vitamin B12 deficiency anemia

SBQ 6

A 75-year-old woman presents to the clinic with fatigue, pallor, and glossitis. She has a history of atrophic gastritis and autoimmune thyroiditis. Her complete blood count shows a hemoglobin of 8.5 g/dL, a mean corpuscular volume (MCV) of 102 fL, and a red cell distribution width (RDW) of 17%. Her serum folate level is low and her serum vitamin B12 level is normal. Her peripheral blood smear shows macrocytic (large) and oval-shaped red blood cells and hypersegmented neutrophils. What is the most likely type of anemia in this patient?
a) Iron deficiency anemia
b) Anemia of chronic disease
c) Thalassemia
d) Sideroblastic anemia
e) Folate deficiency anemia

SBQ 7

A 15-year-old boy presents to the clinic with fatigue, pallor, and splenomegaly. He has a history of sickle cell disease and recurrent vaso-occlusive crises. His complete blood count shows a hemoglobin of 7.0 g/dL, a mean corpuscular volume (MCV) of 88 fL, and a red cell distribution width (RDW) of 20%. His serum iron level is normal, his total iron-binding capacity (TIBC) is normal, and his ferritin level is normal. His peripheral blood smear shows sickle-shaped red blood cells and Howell-Jolly bodies. What is the most likely type of anemia in this patient?

a) Iron deficiency anemia
b) Anemia of chronic disease
c) Thalassemia
d) Sideroblastic anemia
e) Hemolytic anemia

SBQ 8

A 65-year-old woman presents to the clinic with fatigue, pallor, and bruising. She has a history of hypertension and diabetes mellitus. Her complete blood count shows a hemoglobin of 9.0 g/dL, a mean corpuscular volume (MCV) of 90 fL, and a red cell distribution width (RDW) of 14%. Her platelet count is 50,000/mm3 and her white blood cell count is 3,000/mm3. Her serum iron level is normal, her total iron-binding capacity (TIBC) is normal, and her ferritin level is normal. Her bone marrow biopsy shows hypocellularity and increased fat. What is the most likely type of anemia in this patient?
a) Iron deficiency anemia
b) Anemia of chronic disease
c) Thalassemia
d) Sideroblastic anemia
e) Aplastic anemia

SBQ 9

A 35-year-old man presents to the clinic with fatigue, pallor, and leg ulcers. He has a history of glucose-6-phosphate dehydrogenase (G6PD) deficiency and recurrent hemolytic episodes. His complete blood count shows a hemoglobin of 8.5 g/dL, a mean corpuscular volume (MCV) of 92 fL, and a red cell distribution width (RDW) of 19%. His serum iron level is normal, his total iron-binding capacity (TIBC) is normal, and his ferritin level is normal. His peripheral blood smear shows bite cells and Heinz bodies. What is the most likely type of anemia in this patient?
a) Iron deficiency anemia
b) Anemia of chronic disease
c) Thalassemia
d) Sideroblastic anemia
e) Hemolytic anemia

SBQ 10

A 45-year-old woman presents to the clinic with fatigue, pallor, and angular cheilitis. She has a history of celiac disease and gluten-free diet. Her complete blood count shows a hemoglobin of 9.5 g/dL, a mean corpuscular volume (MCV) of 78 fL, and a red cell distribution width (RDW) of 16%. Her serum iron level is low, her total iron-binding capacity (TIBC) is high, and her ferritin level is low. Her serum vitamin B12 level is normal and her serum folate level is low. What is the most likely type of anemia in this patient?
a) Iron deficiency anemia
b) Anemia of chronic disease
c) Thalassemia

d) Sideroblastic anemia
e) Folate deficiency anemia
SBQ 11
A 55-year-old man presents to the clinic with fatigue, pallor, and glossitis.
He has a history of pernicious anemia and gastric bypass surgery. His
complete blood count shows a hemoglobin of 8.0 g/dL, a mean corpuscular
volume (MCV) of 112 fL, and a red cell distribution width (RDW) of 18%. His
serum vitamin B12 level is low, and his serum folate level is normal. His
peripheral blood smear shows macrocytic (large) and oval-shaped red blood
cells and hypersegmented neutrophils. What is the most likely type of
anemia in this patient?
a) Iron deficiency anemia
b) Anemia of chronic disease
c) Thalassemia
d) Sideroblastic anemia
e) Vitamin B12 deficiency anemia
SBQ 12
A 65-year-old woman presents to the clinic with fatigue, pallor, and
petechiae. She has a history of hypertension and diabetes mellitus. Her
complete blood count shows a hemoglobin of 9.0 g/dL, a mean corpuscular
volume (MCV) of 90 fL, and a red cell distribution width (RDW) of 14%. Her
platelet count is 20,000/mm3 and her white blood cell count is 2,000/mm3.
Her serum iron level is normal, her total iron-binding capacity (TIBC) is
normal, and her ferritin level is normal. Her bone marrow biopsy shows
increased blasts. What is the most likely type of anemia in this patient?
a) Iron deficiency anemia
b) Anemia of chronic disease
c) Thalassemia
d) Sideroblastic anemia
e) Aplastic anemia
SBQ 13
A 25-year-old man presents to the clinic with fatigue, pallor, and dark urine.
He has a history of hereditary spherocytosis and splenectomy. His complete
blood count shows a hemoglobin of 9.5 g/dL, a mean corpuscular volume
(MCV) of 100 fL, and a red cell distribution width (RDW) of 18%. His serum
iron level is normal, his total iron-binding capacity (TIBC) is normal, and his
ferritin level is normal. His peripheral blood smear shows spherocytes and
polychromasia. What is the most likely type of anemia in this patient?
a) Iron deficiency anemia
b) Anemia of chronic disease
c) Thalassemia
d) Sideroblastic anemia
e) Hemolytic anemia

SBQ 14

A 35-year-old woman presents to the clinic with fatigue, pallor, and menorrhagia. She has a history of iron deficiency anemia and oral iron supplementation. Her complete blood count shows a hemoglobin of 10.0 g/dL, a mean corpuscular volume (MCV) of 74 fL, and a red cell distribution width (RDW) of 19%. Her serum iron level is low, her total iron-binding capacity (TIBC) is high, and her ferritin level is low. Her serum vitamin B12 level is normal, and her serum folate level is normal. What is the most likely cause of her anemia?

a) Blood loss

b) Dietary deficiency

c) Malabsorption

d) Increased demand

e) Impaired utilization

SBQ 15

A 45-year-old man presents to the clinic with fatigue, pallor, and glossitis. He has a history of atrophic gastritis and autoimmune thyroiditis. His complete blood count shows a hemoglobin of 9.0 g/dL, a mean corpuscular volume (MCV) of 102 fL, and a red cell distribution width (RDW) of 17%. His serum folate level is low and his serum vitamin B12 level is normal. His peripheral blood smear shows macrocytic (large) and oval-shaped red blood cells and hypersegmented neutrophils. What is the most likely type of anemia in this patient?

a) Iron deficiency anemia

b) Anemia of chronic disease

c) Thalassemia

d) Sideroblastic anemia

e) Folate deficiency anemia

SBQ 16

A 55-year-old woman presents to the clinic with fatigue, pallor, and bruising. She has a history of hypertension and diabetes mellitus. Her complete blood count shows a hemoglobin of 9.0 g/dL, a mean corpuscular volume (MCV) of 90 fL, and a red cell distribution width (RDW) of 14%. Her platelet count is 50,000/mm3 and her white blood cell count is 3,000/mm3. Her serum iron level is normal, her total iron-binding capacity (TIBC) is normal, and her ferritin level is normal. Her bone marrow biopsy shows hypocellularity and increased fat. What is the most likely type of anemia in this patient?

a) Iron deficiency anemia

b) Anemia of chronic disease

c) Thalassemia

d) Sideroblastic anemia

e) Aplastic anemia

SBQ 17

A 65-year-old man presents to the clinic with fatigue, pallor, and leg ulcers. He has a history of glucose-6-phosphate dehydrogenase (G6PD) deficiency and recurrent hemolytic episodes. His complete blood count shows a hemoglobin of 8.5 g/dL, a mean corpuscular volume (MCV) of 92 fL, and a red cell distribution width (RDW) of 19%. His serum iron level is normal, his total iron-binding capacity (TIBC) is normal, and his ferritin level is normal. His peripheral blood smear shows bite cells and Heinz bodies. What is the most likely type of anemia in this patient?
a) Iron deficiency anemia
b) Anemia of chronic disease
c) Thalassemia
d) Sideroblastic anemia
e) Hemolytic anemia

SBQ 18

A 25-year-old woman presents to the clinic with fever, sore throat, and lymphadenopathy. Her complete blood count shows a white blood cell count of 15,000/mm3, with 80% lymphocytes, 15% neutrophils, 3% monocytes, 1% eosinophils, and 1% basophils. Her peripheral blood smear shows atypical lymphocytes with abundant cytoplasm and irregular nuclei. What is the most likely diagnosis in this patient?
a) Acute lymphoblastic leukemia
b) Chronic lymphocytic leukemia
c) Infectious mononucleosis
d) Lymphoma
e) Systemic lupus erythematosus

SBQ 19

A 35-year-old man presents to the clinic with fatigue, weight loss, and night sweats. He has a history of tuberculosis and HIV infection. His complete blood count shows a white blood cell count of 3,000/mm3, with 40% lymphocytes, 40% neutrophils, 15% monocytes, 4% eosinophils, and 1% basophils. His peripheral blood smear shows acid-fast bacilli. What is the most likely diagnosis in this patient?
a) Acute myeloid leukemia
b) Chronic myeloid leukemia
c) Disseminated tuberculosis
d) Hodgkin lymphoma
e) Non-Hodgkin lymphoma

SBQ 20

A 45-year-old woman presents to the clinic with recurrent infections, eczema, and asthma. She has a history of allergic rhinitis and food allergies. Her complete blood count shows a white blood cell count of 12,000/mm3, with 50% lymphocytes, 40% neutrophils, 5% monocytes, 4% eosinophils, and

1% basophils. Her peripheral blood smear shows eosinophilia. What is the most likely diagnosis in this patient?
a) Acute eosinophilic leukemia
b) Chronic eosinophilic leukemia
c) Eosinophilic granulomatosis with polyangiitis
d) Hypereosinophilic syndrome
e) Parasitic infection

SBQ 21

A 65-year-old man presents to the clinic with fatigue, weight loss, and night sweats. He has a history of chronic lymphocytic leukemia and is on watchful waiting. His complete blood count shows a white blood cell count of 80,000/mm3, with 90% lymphocytes, 5% neutrophils, 3% monocytes, 1% eosinophils, and 1% basophils. His peripheral blood smear shows small, mature lymphocytes with a narrow rim of cytoplasm and a dense nucleus. What is the most likely complication of his condition?
a) Autoimmune hemolytic anemia
b) Hyperviscosity syndrome
c) Infection
d) Richter transformation
e) Tumor lysis syndrome

SBQ 22

A 35-year-old woman presents to the clinic with recurrent infections, eczema, and asthma. She has a history of allergic rhinitis and food allergies. Her complete blood count shows a white blood cell count of 12,000/mm3, with 50% lymphocytes, 40% neutrophils, 5% monocytes, 4% eosinophils, and 1% basophils. Her peripheral blood smear shows eosinophilia. What is the most likely diagnosis in this patient?
a) Acute eosinophilic leukemia
b) Chronic eosinophilic leukemia
c) Eosinophilic granulomatosis with polyangiitis
d) Hypereosinophilic syndrome
e) Parasitic infection

SBQ 23

A 45-year-old man presents to the clinic with fatigue, weight loss, and night sweats. He has a history of rheumatoid arthritis and chronic kidney disease. His complete blood count shows a white blood cell count of 10,000/mm3, with 60% neutrophils, 30% lymphocytes, 5% monocytes, 3% eosinophils, and 2% basophils. His serum uric acid level is high and his serum creatinine level is high. His peripheral blood smear shows neutrophilia. What is the most likely diagnosis in this patient?
a) Acute myeloid leukemia
b) Chronic myeloid leukemia
c) Gout
d) Polycythemia vera

e) Renal failure
SBQ 24
A 55-year-old woman presents to the clinic with fatigue, pallor, and petechiae. She has a history of hypertension and diabetes mellitus. Her complete blood count shows a white blood cell count of 3,000/mm3, with 40% lymphocytes, 40% neutrophils, 15% monocytes, 4% eosinophils, and 1% basophils. Her platelet count is 50,000/mm3 and her hemoglobin is 9.0 g/dL. Her peripheral blood smear shows pancytopenia. What is the most likely diagnosis in this patient?
a) Aplastic anemia
b) Disseminated intravascular coagulation
c) Myelodysplastic syndrome
d) Paroxysmal nocturnal hemoglobinuria
e) Systemic lupus erythematosus
SBQ 25
A 25-year-old man presents to the clinic with fever, night sweats, and weight loss. He has a history of Down syndrome and no other medical problems. His complete blood count shows a white blood cell count of 100,000/mm3, with 90% blasts, 5% lymphocytes, 3% neutrophils, 1% monocytes, and 1% eosinophils. His peripheral blood smear shows large, immature cells with high nuclear-to-cytoplasmic ratio and prominent nucleoli. What is the most likely diagnosis in this patient?
a) Acute lymphoblastic leukemia
b) Acute myeloid leukemia
c) Chronic lymphocytic leukemia
d) Chronic myeloid leukemia
e) Hairy cell leukemia
SBQ 26
A 35-year-old woman presents to the clinic with fatigue, bruising, and lymphadenopathy. She has a history of autoimmune hemolytic anemia and is on prednisone. Her complete blood count shows a white blood cell count of 20,000/mm3, with 80% lymphocytes, 10% neutrophils, 5% monocytes, 3% eosinophils, and 2% basophils. Her peripheral blood smear shows small, mature lymphocytes with a narrow rim of cytoplasm and a dense nucleus. What is the most likely diagnosis in this patient?
a) Acute lymphoblastic leukemia
b) Acute myeloid leukemia
c) Chronic lymphocytic leukemia
d) Chronic myeloid leukemia
e) Hairy cell leukemia
SBQ 27
A 45-year-old man presents to the clinic with fatigue, weight loss, and night sweats. He has a history of chronic hepatitis C infection and is on antiviral therapy. His complete blood count shows a white blood cell count of

15,000/mm3, with 60% lymphocytes, 30% neutrophils, 5% monocytes, 3% eosinophils, and 2% basophils. His peripheral blood smear shows hairy cells, which are lymphocytes with cytoplasmic projections. What is the most likely diagnosis in this patient?
a) Acute lymphoblastic leukemia
b) Acute myeloid leukemia
c) Chronic lymphocytic leukemia
d) Chronic myeloid leukemia
e) Hairy cell leukemia

SBQ 28

A 25-year-old man presents to the clinic with fever, night sweats, and weight loss. He has a history of Down syndrome and no other medical problems. His complete blood count shows a white blood cell count of 100,000/mm3, with 90% blasts, 5% lymphocytes, 3% neutrophils, 1% monocytes, and 1% eosinophils. His peripheral blood smear shows large, immature cells with high nuclear-to-cytoplasmic ratio and prominent nucleoli. What is the most likely diagnosis in this patient?
a) Acute lymphoblastic leukemia
b) Acute myeloid leukemia
c) Chronic lymphocytic leukemia
d) Chronic myeloid leukemia
e) Hairy cell leukemia

SBQ 29

A 35-year-old woman presents to the clinic with fatigue, bruising, and lymphadenopathy. She has a history of autoimmune hemolytic anemia and is on prednisone. Her complete blood count shows a white blood cell count of 20,000/mm3, with 80% lymphocytes, 10% neutrophils, 5% monocytes, 3% eosinophils, and 2% basophils. Her peripheral blood smear shows small, mature lymphocytes with a narrow rim of cytoplasm and a dense nucleus. What is the most likely diagnosis in this patient?
a) Acute lymphoblastic leukemia
b) Acute myeloid leukemia
c) Chronic lymphocytic leukemia
d) Chronic myeloid leukemia
e) Hairy cell leukemia

SBQ 30

A 45-year-old man presents to the clinic with fatigue, weight loss, and night sweats. He has a history of chronic hepatitis C infection and is on antiviral therapy. His complete blood count shows a white blood cell count of 15,000/mm3, with 60% lymphocytes, 30% neutrophils, 5% monocytes, 3% eosinophils, and 2% basophils. His peripheral blood smear shows hairy cells, which are lymphocytes with cytoplasmic projections. What is the most likely diagnosis in this patient?
a) Acute lymphoblastic leukemia

b) Acute myeloid leukemia
c) Chronic lymphocytic leukemia
d) Chronic myeloid leukemia
e) Hairy cell leukemia

SBQ 31

A 55-year-old woman presents to the clinic with fatigue, pallor, and petechiae. She has a history of hypertension and diabetes mellitus. Her complete blood count shows a white blood cell count of 3,000/mm3, with 40% lymphocytes, 40% neutrophils, 15% monocytes, 4% eosinophils, and 1% basophils. Her platelet count is 50,000/mm3 and her hemoglobin is 9.0 g/dL. Her peripheral blood smear shows pancytopenia. What is the most likely diagnosis in this patient?

a) Aplastic anemia
b) Disseminated intravascular coagulation
c) Myelodysplastic syndrome
d) Paroxysmal nocturnal hemoglobinuria
e) Systemic lupus erythematosus

SBQ 32

A 65-year-old man presents to the clinic with fatigue, weight loss, and splenomegaly. He has a history of gout and is on allopurinol. His complete blood count shows a white blood cell count of 200,000/mm3, with 50% neutrophils, 30% lymphocytes, 10% monocytes, 5% eosinophils, and 5% basophils. His peripheral blood smear shows basophilia and immature myeloid cells. What is the most likely diagnosis in this patient?

a) Acute lymphoblastic leukemia
b) Acute myeloid leukemia
c) Chronic lymphocytic leukemia
d) Chronic myeloid leukemia
e) Hairy cell leukemia

SBQ 33

A 30-year-old woman presents to the clinic with painless swelling of the neck, axillary, and inguinal lymph nodes. She also reports fever, night sweats, weight loss, and itching. Her complete blood count shows a normal hemoglobin, white blood cell count, and platelet count. Her peripheral blood smear shows no abnormal cells. Her lymph node biopsy shows Reed-Sternberg cells, which are large, binucleated cells with prominent nucleoli. What is the most likely diagnosis in this patient?

a) Hodgkin lymphoma
b) Non-Hodgkin lymphoma
c) Acute lymphoblastic leukemia
d) Chronic lymphocytic leukemia
e) Infectious mononucleosis

SBQ 34

A 50-year-old man presents to the clinic with fatigue, anemia, and splenomegaly. He has a history of hepatitis C infection and is on antiviral therapy. His complete blood count shows a hemoglobin of 9 g/dL, a white blood cell count of 4,000/mm3, and a platelet count of 100,000/mm3. His peripheral blood smear shows small, mature lymphocytes with irregular nuclei and cytoplasmic projections. His serum protein electrophoresis shows a monoclonal spike of IgM. His bone marrow biopsy shows infiltration of lymphoplasmacytic cells. What is the most likely diagnosis in this patient?
a) Hodgkin lymphoma
b) Non-Hodgkin lymphoma
c) Acute lymphoblastic leukemia
d) Chronic lymphocytic leukemia
e) Infectious mononucleosis

SBQ 35

A 40-year-old woman presents to the clinic with abdominal pain, weight loss, and night sweats. She has a history of celiac disease and is on a gluten-free diet. Her complete blood count shows a hemoglobin of 10 g/dL, a white blood cell count of 6,000/mm3, and a platelet count of 150,000/mm3. Her peripheral blood smear shows no abnormal cells. Her abdominal CT scan shows multiple enlarged mesenteric lymph nodes. Her lymph node biopsy shows small, cleaved cells with irregular nuclei and scant cytoplasm. Her immunohistochemistry shows positive staining for CD20, CD10, and BCL-6. What is the most likely diagnosis in this patient?
a) Hodgkin lymphoma
b) Non-Hodgkin lymphoma
c) Acute lymphoblastic leukemia
d) Chronic lymphocytic leukemia
e) Infectious mononucleosis

SBQ 36

A 60-year-old man presents to the clinic with cough, dyspnea, and chest pain. He has a history of smoking and chronic obstructive pulmonary disease. His complete blood count shows a hemoglobin of 11 g/dL, a white blood cell count of 8,000/mm3, and a platelet count of 200,000/mm3. His peripheral blood smear shows no abnormal cells. His chest X-ray shows a large mediastinal mass. His lymph node biopsy shows large, atypical cells with multilobed nuclei and prominent nucleoli. His immunohistochemistry shows positive staining for CD30, CD15, and PAX5. What is the most likely diagnosis in this patient?
a) Hodgkin lymphoma
b) Non-Hodgkin lymphoma
c) Acute lymphoblastic leukemia
d) Chronic lymphocytic leukemia
e) Infectious mononucleosis

SBQ 37

A 70-year-old woman presents to the clinic with fatigue, anemia, and lymphadenopathy. She has a history of rheumatoid arthritis and is on methotrexate and prednisone. Her complete blood count shows a hemoglobin of 9 g/dL, a white blood cell count of 10,000/mm3, and a platelet count of 150,000/mm3. Her peripheral blood smear shows small, mature lymphocytes with round nuclei and clumped chromatin. Her lymph node biopsy shows diffuse infiltration of small, mature lymphocytes with round nuclei and clumped chromatin. Her immunohistochemistry shows positive staining for CD20, CD5, and CD23. What is the most likely diagnosis in this patient?
a) Hodgkin lymphoma
b) Non-Hodgkin lymphoma
c) Acute lymphoblastic leukemia
d) Chronic lymphocytic leukemia
e) Infectious mononucleosis

SBQ 38

A 45-year-old man presents to the clinic with headache, dizziness, and blurred vision. He has a history of smoking and hypertension. His complete blood count shows a hemoglobin of 20 g/dL, a hematocrit of 60%, and a red blood cell count of 7 million/mm3. His serum erythropoietin level is low. What is the most likely diagnosis in this patient?
a) Primary polycythemia
b) Secondary polycythemia due to hypoxia
c) Secondary polycythemia due to erythropoietin-producing tumor
d) Secondary polycythemia due to dehydration
e) Secondary polycythemia due to testosterone therapy

SBQ 39

A 55-year-old woman presents to the clinic with fatigue, dyspnea, and cyanosis. She has a history of chronic obstructive pulmonary disease (COPD) and oxygen therapy. Her complete blood count shows a hemoglobin of 18 g/dL, a hematocrit of 54%, and a red blood cell count of 6 million/mm3. Her serum erythropoietin level is high. What is the most likely diagnosis in this patient?
a) Primary polycythemia
b) Secondary polycythemia due to hypoxia
c) Secondary polycythemia due to erythropoietin-producing tumor
d) Secondary polycythemia due to dehydration
e) Secondary polycythemia due to testosterone therapy

SBQ 40

A 65-year-old man presents to the clinic with abdominal pain, weight loss, and night sweats. He has a history of renal cell carcinoma and nephrectomy. His complete blood count shows a hemoglobin of 19 g/dL, a hematocrit of

57%, and a red blood cell count of 6.5 million/mm3. His serum erythropoietin level is high. What is the most likely diagnosis in this patient?
a) Primary polycythemia
b) Secondary polycythemia due to hypoxia
c) Secondary polycythemia due to erythropoietin-producing tumor
d) Secondary polycythemia due to dehydration
e) Secondary polycythemia due to testosterone therapy

SBQ 41

A 75-year-old woman presents to the clinic with weakness, confusion, and constipation. She has a history of diabetes mellitus and diuretic therapy. Her complete blood count shows a hemoglobin of 17 g/dL, a hematocrit of 51%, and a red blood cell count of 5.5 million/mm3. Her serum erythropoietin level is normal. What is the most likely diagnosis in this patient?
a) Primary polycythemia
b) Secondary polycythemia due to hypoxia
c) Secondary polycythemia due to erythropoietin-producing tumor
d) Secondary polycythemia due to dehydration
e) Secondary polycythemia due to testosterone therapy

SBQ 42

A 85-year-old man presents to the clinic with erectile dysfunction, mood swings, and decreased muscle mass. He has a history of hypogonadism and testosterone therapy. His complete blood count shows a hemoglobin of 16 g/dL, a hematocrit of 48%, and a red blood cell count of 5 million/mm3. His serum erythropoietin level is normal. What is the most likely diagnosis in this patient?
a) Primary polycythemia
b) Secondary polycythemia due to hypoxia
c) Secondary polycythemia due to erythropoietin-producing tumor
d) Secondary polycythemia due to dehydration
e) Secondary polycythemia due to testosterone therapy

SBQ 43

A 55-year-old man presents to the clinic with bone pain, anemia, and renal insufficiency. He has a history of monoclonal gammopathy of undetermined significance (MGUS) and is on watchful waiting. His serum protein electrophoresis shows a monoclonal spike of IgG kappa. His urine protein electrophoresis shows Bence Jones protein. His bone marrow biopsy shows 40% plasma cells. What is the most likely diagnosis in this patient?
a) Multiple myeloma
b) Waldenstrom macroglobulinemia
c) Primary amyloidosis
d) Heavy chain disease
e) Plasmacytoma

SBQ 44

A 65-year-old woman presents to the clinic with fatigue, bruising, and recurrent infections. She has a history of multiple myeloma and is on chemotherapy. Her complete blood count shows a hemoglobin of 8 g/dL, a white blood cell count of 2,000/mm3, and a platelet count of 50,000/mm3. Her serum protein electrophoresis shows a monoclonal spike of IgA lambda. Her urine protein electrophoresis shows Bence Jones protein. Her bone marrow biopsy shows 60% plasma cells. What is the most likely complication of her condition?
a) Hyperviscosity syndrome
b) Amyloidosis
c) Hypercalcemia
d) Tumor lysis syndrome
e) Autoimmune hemolytic anemia

SBQ 45

A 75-year-old man presents to the clinic with back pain, constipation, and confusion. He has a history of hypertension and diabetes mellitus. His complete blood count shows a hemoglobin of 10 g/dL, a white blood cell count of 5,000/mm3, and a platelet count of 150,000/mm3. His serum protein electrophoresis shows a monoclonal spike of IgG lambda. His urine protein electrophoresis shows Bence Jones protein. His bone marrow biopsy shows 30% plasma cells. His serum calcium level is 12 mg/dL. What is the most likely cause of his hypercalcemia?
a) Bone resorption due to osteoclast activation by cytokines from plasma cells
b) Renal failure due to light chain cast nephropathy
c) Dehydration due to vomiting, diarrhea, or diuretic therapy
d) Parathyroid hormone-related peptide (PTHrP) secretion by plasma cells
e) Vitamin D intoxication due to excessive supplementation

SBQ 46

A 85-year-old woman presents to the clinic with blurred vision, headache, and bleeding gums. She has a history of multiple myeloma and is on chemotherapy. Her complete blood count shows a hemoglobin of 9 g/dL, a white blood cell count of 4,000/mm3, and a platelet count of 100,000/mm3. Her serum protein electrophoresis shows a monoclonal spike of IgM kappa. Her urine protein electrophoresis shows Bence Jones protein. Her bone marrow biopsy shows 50% plasma cells. Her serum viscosity is 6 centipoise (normal range: 1.4 to 1.8 centipoise). What is the most likely diagnosis in this patient?
a) Hyperviscosity syndrome
b) Amyloidosis
c) Hypercalcemia
d) Tumor lysis syndrome
e) Autoimmune hemolytic anemia

SBQ 47

A 95-year-old man presents to the clinic with fatigue, anemia, and renal insufficiency. He has a history of multiple myeloma and is on chemotherapy. His complete blood count shows a hemoglobin of 7 g/dL, a white blood cell count of 3,000/mm3, and a platelet count of 80,000/mm3. His serum protein electrophoresis shows a monoclonal spike of IgG kappa. His urine protein electrophoresis shows Bence Jones protein. His bone marrow biopsy shows 70% plasma cells. His serum uric acid level is 12 mg/dL. His serum creatinine level is 3 mg/dL. What is the most likely cause of his renal failure?
a) Light chain cast nephropathy
b) Amyloidosis
c) Hypercalcemia
d) Tumor lysis syndrome
e) Glomerulonephritis

SBQ 48

A 25-year-old woman presents to the clinic with easy bruising, epistaxis, and menorrhagia. She has no history of bleeding disorders or medications. Her complete blood count shows a normal hemoglobin, white blood cell count, and platelet count. Her bleeding time is prolonged, but her prothrombin time and activated partial thromboplastin time are normal. Her platelet aggregation test shows normal response to ristocetin, but impaired response to ADP, collagen, and epinephrine. What is the most likely diagnosis in this patient?
a) Glanzmann thrombasthenia
b) Bernard-Soulier syndrome
c) von Willebrand disease
d) Aspirin-induced platelet dysfunction
e) Uremic platelet dysfunction

SBQ 49

A 35-year-old man presents to the clinic with recurrent episodes of thrombosis, including deep vein thrombosis, pulmonary embolism, and stroke. He has no history of trauma, surgery, or malignancy. His complete blood count shows a normal hemoglobin, white blood cell count, and platelet count. His prothrombin time and activated partial thromboplastin time are normal. His platelet aggregation test shows normal response to all agonists. His plasma serotonin level is elevated. What is the most likely diagnosis in this patient?
a) Essential thrombocythemia
b) Polycythemia vera
c) Heparin-induced thrombocytopenia
d) Antiphospholipid syndrome
e) Carcinoid syndrome

SBQ 50

A 45-year-old woman presents to the clinic with petechiae, purpura, and gingival bleeding. She has a history of systemic lupus erythematosus and is on prednisone and hydroxychloroquine. Her complete blood count shows a normal hemoglobin, white blood cell count, and red blood cell morphology. Her platelet count is 20,000/mm3. Her prothrombin time and activated partial thromboplastin time are normal. Her peripheral blood smear shows no platelet clumps or schistocytes. Her direct and indirect antiglobulin tests are negative. Her platelet-associated IgG level is elevated. What is the most likely diagnosis in this patient?

a) Immune thrombocytopenic purpura

b) Thrombotic thrombocytopenic purpura

c) Disseminated intravascular coagulation

d) Hemolytic uremic syndrome

e) Drug-induced thrombocytopenia

SBQ 51

A 20-year-old man presents to the clinic with recurrent episodes of epistaxis, gingival bleeding, and hematuria. He has a history of mild anemia and easy bruising since childhood. His complete blood count shows a normal hemoglobin, white blood cell count, and platelet count. His bleeding time is prolonged, but his prothrombin time and activated partial thromboplastin time are normal. His platelet aggregation test shows normal response to ristocetin, but absent response to ADP, collagen, epinephrine, and arachidonic acid. What is the most likely diagnosis in this patient?

a) Glanzmann thrombasthenia

b) Bernard-Soulier syndrome

c) von Willebrand disease

d) Aspirin-induced platelet dysfunction

e) Uremic platelet dysfunction

SBQ 52

A 30-year-old woman presents to the clinic with petechiae, purpura, and ecchymoses. She has no history of bleeding disorders or medications. Her complete blood count shows a normal hemoglobin, white blood cell count, and red blood cell morphology. Her platelet count is 10,000/mm3. Her prothrombin time and activated partial thromboplastin time are normal. Her peripheral blood smear shows no platelet clumps or schistocytes. Her direct and indirect antiglobulin tests are negative. Her platelet-associated IgG level is normal. What is the most likely diagnosis in this patient?

a) Immune thrombocytopenic purpura

b) Thrombotic thrombocytopenic purpura

c) Disseminated intravascular coagulation

d) Hemolytic uremic syndrome

e) Drug-induced thrombocytopenia

SBQ 53
A 40-year-old man presents to the clinic with fatigue, pallor, and dyspnea. He has a history of chronic renal failure and is on hemodialysis. His complete blood count shows a hemoglobin of 8 g/dL, a white blood cell count of 6,000/mm3, and a platelet count of 150,000/mm3. His bleeding time is prolonged, but his prothrombin time and activated partial thromboplastin time are normal. His platelet aggregation test shows impaired response to all agonists. His serum creatinine level is 5 mg/dL. What is the most likely cause of his bleeding tendency?
a) Glanzmann thrombasthenia
b) Bernard-Soulier syndrome
c) von Willebrand disease
d) Aspirin-induced platelet dysfunction
e) Uremic platelet dysfunction

SBQ 54
A 50-year-old woman presents to the clinic with recurrent episodes of thrombosis, including deep vein thrombosis, pulmonary embolism, and stroke. She has no history of trauma, surgery, or malignancy. Her complete blood count shows a normal hemoglobin, white blood cell count, and red blood cell morphology. Her platelet count is 600,000/mm3. Her prothrombin time and activated partial thromboplastin time are normal. Her platelet aggregation test shows normal response to all agonists. Her bone marrow biopsy shows increased number and size of megakaryocytes. What is the most likely diagnosis in this patient?
a) Essential thrombocythemia
b) Polycythemia vera
c) Heparin-induced thrombocytopenia
d) Antiphospholipid syndrome
e) Carcinoid syndrome

SBQ 55
A 60-year-old man presents to the clinic with easy bruising, epistaxis, and hematuria. He has a history of coronary artery disease and is on aspirin and clopidogrel. His complete blood count shows a normal hemoglobin, white blood cell count, and platelet count. His bleeding time is prolonged, but his prothrombin time and activated partial thromboplastin time are normal. His platelet aggregation test shows normal response to ristocetin, but reduced response to ADP, collagen, epinephrine, and arachidonic acid. What is the most likely cause of his bleeding tendency?
a) Glanzmann thrombasthenia
b) Bernard-Soulier syndrome
c) von Willebrand disease
d) Aspirin-induced platelet dysfunction
e) Uremic platelet dysfunction

SBQ 56

A 20-year-old woman presents to the clinic with heavy menstrual bleeding, easy bruising, and frequent nosebleeds. She has a family history of bleeding disorders. Her complete blood count shows a normal hemoglobin, white blood cell count, and platelet count. Her bleeding time is prolonged, but her prothrombin time and activated partial thromboplastin time are normal. Her von Willebrand factor antigen and activity levels are low. What is the most likely diagnosis in this patient?

a) Hemophilia A

b) Hemophilia B

c) von Willebrand disease

d) Factor XIII deficiency

e) Glanzmann thrombasthenia

SBQ 57

A 30-year-old man presents to the clinic with recurrent episodes of deep vein thrombosis and pulmonary embolism. He has no history of trauma, surgery, or malignancy. His complete blood count shows a normal hemoglobin, white blood cell count, and platelet count. His prothrombin time and activated partial thromboplastin time are normal. His plasma D-dimer level is elevated. His genetic testing shows a mutation in the factor V gene that renders it resistant to the inactivation by activated protein C. What is the most likely diagnosis in this patient?

a) Factor V Leiden

b) Protein C deficiency

c) Protein S deficiency

d) Antithrombin deficiency

e) Prothrombin gene mutation

SBQ 58

A 40-year-old woman presents to the clinic with petechiae, purpura, and bleeding gums. She has a history of systemic lupus erythematosus and is on prednisone and hydroxychloroquine. Her complete blood count shows a normal hemoglobin, white blood cell count, and red blood cell morphology. Her platelet count is 20,000/mm3. Her prothrombin time and activated partial thromboplastin time are normal. Her peripheral blood smear shows no platelet clumps or schistocytes. Her direct and indirect antiglobulin tests are negative. Her platelet-associated IgG level is elevated. What is the most likely diagnosis in this patient?

a) Immune thrombocytopenic purpura

b) Thrombotic thrombocytopenic purpura

c) Disseminated intravascular coagulation

d) Hemolytic uremic syndrome

e) Drug-induced thrombocytopenia

SBQ 59

A 50-year-old man presents to the clinic with fatigue, pallor, and dyspnea. He has a history of chronic renal failure and is on hemodialysis. His complete blood count shows a hemoglobin of 8 g/dL, a white blood cell count of 6,000/mm3, and a platelet count of 150,000/mm3. His bleeding time is prolonged, but his prothrombin time and activated partial thromboplastin time are normal. His platelet aggregation test shows impaired response to all agonists. His serum creatinine level is 5 mg/dL. What is the most likely cause of his bleeding tendency?

a) Glanzmann thrombasthenia

b) Bernard-Soulier syndrome

c) von Willebrand disease

d) Aspirin-induced platelet dysfunction

e) Uremic platelet dysfunction

SBQ 60

A 60-year-old woman presents to the clinic with recurrent episodes of thrombosis, including deep vein thrombosis, pulmonary embolism, and stroke. She has no history of trauma, surgery, or malignancy. Her complete blood count shows a normal hemoglobin, white blood cell count, and platelet count. Her prothrombin time and activated partial thromboplastin time are normal. Her plasma D-dimer level is elevated. Her anticardiolipin antibody and lupus anticoagulant tests are positive. What is the most likely diagnosis in this patient?

a) Factor V Leiden

b) Protein C deficiency

c) Protein S deficiency

d) Antithrombin deficiency

e) Antiphospholipid syndrome

SBQ 61

A 25-year-old man presents to the clinic with hemarthrosis, muscle hematoma, and prolonged bleeding after minor trauma. He has a family history of bleeding disorders. His complete blood count shows a normal hemoglobin, white blood cell count, and platelet count. His bleeding time is normal, but his prothrombin time is normal, and his activated partial thromboplastin time is prolonged. His factor VIII activity level is low. What is the most likely diagnosis in this patient?

a) Hemophilia A

b) Hemophilia B

c) von Willebrand disease

d) Factor XIII deficiency

e) Glanzmann thrombasthenia

SBQ 62

A 35-year-old woman presents to the clinic with recurrent miscarriages, fetal growth restriction, and placental abruption. She has no history of bleeding

disorders or thrombosis. Her complete blood count shows a normal hemoglobin, white blood cell count, and platelet count. Her prothrombin time and activated partial thromboplastin time are normal. Her plasma D-dimer level is normal. Her anticardiolipin antibody and lupus anticoagulant tests are positive. What is the most likely diagnosis in this patient?
a) Factor V Leiden
b) Protein C deficiency
c) Protein S deficiency
d) Antithrombin deficiency
e) Antiphospholipid syndrome

SBQ 63

A 45-year-old man presents to the clinic with petechiae, purpura, and bleeding from multiple sites. He has a history of sepsis and is on broad-spectrum antibiotics. His complete blood count shows a hemoglobin of 10 g/dL, a white blood cell count of 15,000/mm3, and a platelet count of 50,000/mm3. His prothrombin time and activated partial thromboplastin time are prolonged. His plasma D-dimer level is elevated. His peripheral blood smear shows platelet clumps and schistocytes. His fibrinogen level is low. What is the most likely diagnosis in this patient?
a) Immune thrombocytopenic purpura
b) Thrombotic thrombocytopenic purpura
c) Disseminated intravascular coagulation
d) Hemolytic uremic syndrome
e) Drug-induced thrombocytopenia

SBQ 64

A 55-year-old woman presents to the clinic with fatigue, pallor, and dyspnea. She has a history of chronic liver disease and is on anticoagulant therapy. Her complete blood count shows a hemoglobin of 9 g/dL, a white blood cell count of 5,000/mm3, and a platelet count of 100,000/mm3. Her prothrombin time and activated partial thromboplastin time are prolonged. Her plasma D-dimer level is normal. Her peripheral blood smear shows no platelet clumps or schistocytes. Her fibrinogen level is normal. What is the most likely cause of her coagulation abnormality?
a) Glanzmann thrombasthenia
b) Bernard-Soulier syndrome
c) von Willebrand disease
d) Aspirin-induced platelet dysfunction
e) Uremic platelet dysfunction

SBQ 65

A 65-year-old man presents to the clinic with recurrent episodes of deep vein thrombosis and pulmonary embolism. He has a history of trauma, surgery, and malignancy. His complete blood count shows a normal hemoglobin, white blood cell count, and platelet count. His prothrombin time and activated partial thromboplastin time are normal. His plasma D-

dimer level is elevated. His antithrombin activity level is low. What is the most likely diagnosis in this patient?
a) Factor V Leiden
b) Protein C deficiency
c) Protein S deficiency
d) Antithrombin deficiency
e) Antiphospholipid syndrome

SBQ 66

A nurse is preparing to administer a unit of packed red blood cells to a patient with severe anemia. The nurse verifies the patient's identity and blood group with another nurse. The nurse also checks the expiration date and appearance of the blood unit. What else should the nurse do before starting the transfusion?
a) Obtain informed consent from the patient or a legal representative.
b) Administer an antipyretic and an antihistamine to the patient.
c) Flush the intravenous line with normal saline.
e) Record the patient's vital signs and urine output.

SBQ 67

A patient is receiving a unit of fresh frozen plasma to correct a coagulation disorder. The nurse notices that the patient develops urticaria, pruritus, and flushing during the transfusion. The nurse stops the transfusion and notifies the health care provider. The health care provider prescribes diphenhydramine (Benadryl) 25 mg intravenously. How should the nurse administer the medication?
a) Through the same intravenous line as the blood transfusion.
b) Through a separate dedicated intravenous line from the blood transfusion.
c) After diluting the medication with 50 mL of normal saline.
d) After flushing the intravenous line with 10 mL of heparinized saline.
e) Through a separate intravenous line from the blood transfusion

SBQ 68

A patient is receiving a unit of platelets to treat thrombocytopenia. The nurse observes that the patient develops fever, chills, and rigors during the transfusion. The nurse stops the transfusion and notifies the health care provider. The health care provider prescribes acetaminophen (Tylenol) 500 mg orally. What is the most likely cause of the patient's reaction?
a) Acute hemolytic reaction
b) Febrile nonhemolytic reaction
c) Allergic reaction
d) Bacterial contamination
e) Circulatory overload

SBQ 69

A patient is receiving a unit of whole blood to treat severe blood loss after a motor vehicle accident. The nurse monitors the patient closely for any signs of transfusion reactions. The nurse also ensures that the transfusion is completed within how many hours of obtaining the blood unit from the blood bank?

a) 2 hours
b) 4 hours
c) 6 hours
d) 8 hours
e) 10 hours

SBQ 70

A patient is receiving a unit of cryoprecipitate to treat hemophilia A. The nurse explains to the patient that cryoprecipitate is a blood product that contains high concentrations of which coagulation factor?

a) Factor VIII
b) Factor IX
c) Factor X
d) Factor XI
e) Fibrinogen

SBQ 71

A patient is receiving a unit of packed red blood cells to treat severe anemia due to chronic kidney disease. The nurse notices that the patient develops dyspnea, wheezes, and hypoxia during the transfusion. The nurse stops the transfusion and notifies the health care provider. The health care provider prescribes oxygen, epinephrine, and corticosteroids. What is the most likely cause of the patient's reaction?

a) Acute hemolytic reaction
b) Febrile nonhemolytic reaction
c) Allergic reaction
d) Transfusion-related acute lung injury
e) Circulatory overload

SBQ 72

A patient is receiving a unit of fresh frozen plasma to correct a coagulation disorder due to liver cirrhosis. The nurse observes that the patient develops fever, chills, hypotension, and tachycardia during the transfusion. The nurse stops the transfusion and notifies the health care provider. The health care provider orders blood cultures and broad-spectrum antibiotics. What is the most likely cause of the patient's reaction?

a) Acute hemolytic reaction
b) Febrile nonhemolytic reaction
c) Allergic reaction
d) Bacterial contamination
e) Transfusion-associated graft-versus-host disease

SBQ 73

A patient is receiving a unit of platelets to treat thrombocytopenia due to chemotherapy. The nurse checks that the patient's blood group is AB positive and that the platelet unit is O negative. The nurse administers the platelet unit without any complications. Why is it safe to transfuse O negative platelets to an AB positive patient?

a) Because platelets do not have ABO antigens

b) Because platelets do not have Rh antigens

c) Because O negative is the universal donor for platelets

d) Because AB positive is the universal recipient for platelets

e) Because the plasma volume in platelets is negligible

SBQ 74

A patient is receiving a unit of whole blood to treat severe blood loss after a gunshot wound. The nurse ensures that the patient's blood group is B positive and that the blood unit is B positive. The nurse also ensures that the blood unit is compatible with the patient's blood type by performing a crossmatch test. What is the purpose of the crossmatch test?

a) To confirm the patient's blood group

b) To confirm the blood unit's blood group

c) To detect any unexpected antibodies in the patient's plasma

d) To detect any unexpected antibodies in the blood unit's plasma

e) To detect any hemolysis in the patient's red blood cells

SBQ 75

A patient is receiving a unit of cryoprecipitate to treat hemophilia A. The nurse explains to the patient that cryoprecipitate is a blood product that contains high concentrations of factor VIII, as well as fibrinogen, von Willebrand factor, and factor XIII. The nurse also explains that cryoprecipitate is derived from which blood component?

a) Red blood cells

b) Platelets

c) Plasma

d) Granulocytes

e) Stem cells

SBQ 76

A 6-month-old boy is brought to the clinic by his parents, who are concerned about his pale skin and poor feeding. His parents are first cousins and have a family history of anemia. His complete blood count shows a hemoglobin of 6 g/dL, a mean corpuscular volume (MCV) of 60 fL, and a reticulocyte count of 0.5%. His peripheral blood smear shows microcytic, hypochromic red blood cells with target cells and basophilic stippling. His serum iron, total iron-binding capacity, and ferritin levels are normal. What is the most likely diagnosis in this patient?

a) Iron deficiency anemia

b) Thalassemia

c) Sideroblastic anemia
d) Lead poisoning
e) Anemia of chronic disease

SBQ 77

A 4-year-old girl is admitted to the hospital with fever, malaise, and petechiae. She has a history of recurrent infections and easy bruising. Her complete blood count shows a hemoglobin of 8 g/dL, a white blood cell count of 2,000/mm3, and a platelet count of 20,000/mm3. Her peripheral blood smear shows pancytopenia with blasts. Her bone marrow biopsy shows hypercellularity with > 20% blasts. Her immunophenotyping shows positive staining for CD19, CD10, CD34, and TdT. What is the most likely diagnosis in this patient?
a) Acute lymphoblastic leukemia
b) Acute myeloid leukemia
c) Chronic lymphocytic leukemia
d) Chronic myeloid leukemia
e) Lymphoma

SBQ 78

A 10-year-old boy is evaluated for pallor, fatigue, and jaundice. He has a history of neonatal jaundice and splenectomy at age 2. His complete blood count shows a hemoglobin of 9 g/dL, a reticulocyte count of 8%, and a normal white blood cell count and platelet count. His peripheral blood smear shows spherocytes, polychromasia, and Howell-Jolly bodies. His serum bilirubin level is elevated, mainly due to indirect bilirubin. His serum lactate dehydrogenase level is also elevated. His direct antiglobulin test is negative. What is the most likely diagnosis in this patient?
a) Hereditary spherocytosis
b) Autoimmune hemolytic anemia
c) Glucose-6-phosphate dehydrogenase deficiency
d) Sickle cell anemia
e) Thalassemia

SBQ 79

A 2-year-old girl is brought to the clinic by her parents, who are concerned about her recurrent episodes of abdominal pain, swelling, and vomiting. She also has a history of failure to thrive, chronic diarrhea, and recurrent respiratory infections. Her physical examination reveals pallor, hepatosplenomegaly, and skeletal deformities. Her complete blood count shows a hemoglobin of 7 g/dL, a white blood cell count of 15,000/mm3, and a platelet count of 100,000/mm3. Her peripheral blood smear shows normocytic, normochromic red blood cells with vacuoles, and leukocytes with cytoplasmic inclusions. Her serum acid phosphatase level is elevated. What is the most likely diagnosis in this patient?
a) Gaucher disease
b) Niemann-Pick disease

c) Tay-Sachs disease
d) Hurler syndrome
e) Fabry disease

SBQ 80

A 12-year-old boy is referred to the clinic for evaluation of short stature. He has a history of frequent nosebleeds, easy bruising, and prolonged bleeding after dental extraction. His physical examination reveals a height of 140 cm (< 3rd percentile), a weight of 35 kg (10th percentile), and a head circumference of 52 cm (50th percentile). He also has telangiectasias on his lips, tongue, and nasal mucosa. His complete blood count shows a hemoglobin of 10 g/dL, a white blood cell count of 5,000/mm3, and a platelet count of 150,000/mm3. His bleeding time is prolonged, but his prothrombin time and activated partial thromboplastin time are normal. His serum iron, total iron-binding capacity, and ferritin levels are normal. What is the most likely diagnosis in this patient?

a) Hemophilia A
b) Hemophilia B
c) von Willebrand disease
d) Factor XIII deficiency
e) Hereditary hemorrhagic telangiectasia

SBQ 81

A 3-month-old girl is brought to the clinic by her parents, who are concerned about her yellow skin and eyes. She was born at term with no complications. Her parents are of African descent and have no history of blood disorders. Her complete blood count shows a hemoglobin of 7 g/dL, a mean corpuscular volume (MCV) of 90 fL, and a reticulocyte count of 15%. Her peripheral blood smear shows normocytic, normochromic red blood cells with sickle-shaped cells and nucleated red blood cells. Her serum bilirubin level is elevated, mainly due to indirect bilirubin. Her hemoglobin electrophoresis shows hemoglobin S of 85% and hemoglobin F of 15%. What is the most likely diagnosis in this patient?

a) Sickle cell anemia
b) Sickle cell trait
c) Beta thalassemia major
d) Beta thalassemia minor
e) Glucose-6-phosphate dehydrogenase deficiency

SBQ 82

A 6-year-old boy is evaluated for recurrent epistaxis, gingival bleeding, and hematomas. He has a history of prolonged bleeding after circumcision and immunizations. His physical examination reveals multiple ecchymoses and petechiae on his skin and mucous membranes. His complete blood count shows a normal hemoglobin, white blood cell count, and platelet count. His bleeding time is normal, but his prothrombin time is normal, and his

activated partial thromboplastin time is prolonged. His factor VIII activity level is low. What is the most likely diagnosis in this patient?
a) Hemophilia A
b) Hemophilia B
c) von Willebrand disease
d) Factor XIII deficiency
e) Glanzmann thrombasthenia

SBQ 83

A 9-year-old girl is admitted to the hospital with fever, fatigue, and bone pain. She has a history of pallor, easy bruising, and frequent infections. Her complete blood count shows a hemoglobin of 8 g/dL, a white blood cell count of 50,000/mm3, and a platelet count of 50,000/mm3. Her peripheral blood smear shows pancytopenia with blasts. Her bone marrow biopsy shows hypercellularity with > 20% blasts. Her immunophenotyping shows positive staining for CD13, CD33, CD117, and MPO. What is the most likely diagnosis in this patient?
a) Acute lymphoblastic leukemia
b) Acute myeloid leukemia
c) Chronic lymphocytic leukemia
d) Chronic myeloid leukemia
e) Lymphoma

SBQ 84

A 2-year-old boy is brought to the clinic by his parents, who are concerned about his pale skin and poor growth. He was born at term with no complications. His parents are of Southeast Asian descent and have no history of blood disorders. His complete blood count shows a hemoglobin of 6 g/dL, a mean corpuscular volume (MCV) of 60 fL, and a reticulocyte count of 1%. His peripheral blood smear shows microcytic, hypochromic red blood cells with target cells and basophilic stippling. His serum iron, total iron-binding capacity, and ferritin levels are normal. His hemoglobin electrophoresis shows hemoglobin E of 95% and hemoglobin A2 of 5%. What is the most likely diagnosis in this patient?
a) Iron deficiency anemia
b) Thalassemia
c) Sideroblastic anemia
d) Lead poisoning
e) Anemia of chronic disease

SBQ 85

A 7-year-old boy is evaluated for recurrent abdominal pain, joint pain, and priapism. He has a history of neonatal jaundice and splenectomy at age 3. His complete blood count shows a hemoglobin of 8 g/dL, a mean corpuscular volume (MCV) of 90 fL, and a reticulocyte count of 10%. His peripheral blood smear shows normocytic, normochromic red blood cells with sickle-shaped cells and Howell-Jolly bodies. His serum bilirubin level is

elevated, mainly due to indirect bilirubin. His hemoglobin electrophoresis shows hemoglobin S of 60% and hemoglobin C of 40%. What is the most likely diagnosis in this patient?
a) Sickle cell anemia
b) Sickle cell trait
c) Hemoglobin SC disease
d) Hemoglobin C disease
e) Glucose-6-phosphate dehydrogenase deficiency

Section 3
Extended Matching Questions 1-50

This part contains 50 extended matching questions (EMG), which are intended to improve your knowledge of hematology through complicated problem-solving and comprehensive analysis. These questions will challenge you to use your knowledge in an expanded way because they are designed to reflect the complexities of clinical decision-making.

The expanded matching format demands you match a series of options to a list of clinical scenarios, putting your ability to distinguish subtle differences and similarities across various hematological conditions to the test. This activity will help you improve your diagnostic skills and make educated clinical decisions.

This part provides an excellent chance for students to engage with hematology in a manner that encourages critical thinking and accuracy. It is especially useful for individuals studying for higher-level exams or wanting to learn the art of differential diagnosis in hematology.

We hope that the extended matching questions will not only challenge your knowledge but also inspire you to appreciate the hematological sciences' complexity and beauty.

Answers will be found on pages 116 – 128.

EMQ 1

Match each patient with the most likely type of anemia.
1. Iron deficiency anemia.
2. Vitamin B12 deficiency anemia.
3. Folate deficiency anemia.
4. Hereditary spherocytosis.
5. Sickle cell anemia.

A. A 67-year-old man with fatigue, pallor, and macrocytic red blood cells. His serum vitamin B12 level is low.

B. A 45-year-old woman with heavy menstrual bleeding, spoon-shaped nails, and microcytic hypochromic red blood cells. Her serum ferritin level is low.

C. A 32-year-old man with jaundice, splenomegaly, and spherocytic red blood cells. His direct antiglobulin test is negative.

D. A 25-year-old woman with paresthesia, glossitis, and macrocytic red blood cells. Her serum folate level is low.

E. A 21-year-old man with sickle cell disease, vaso-occlusive crisis, and normocytic normochromic red blood cells. His hemoglobin electrophoresis shows hemoglobin S.

EMQ 2

Match each patient with the most likely cause of their anemia.
1. Chronic inflammation.
2. Iron deficiency.
3. Autoimmune gastritis.
4. Dietary deficiency.
5. Autoimmune hemolysis

A. A 72-year-old woman with rheumatoid arthritis, normocytic normochromic anemia, and low serum iron and transferrin levels.

B. A 65-year-old man with gastric adenocarcinoma, microcytic hypochromic anemia, and low serum iron and ferritin levels.

C. A 55-year-old woman with pernicious anemia, macrocytic anemia, and low serum vitamin B12 and intrinsic factor levels.

D. A 35-year-old man with alcoholism, macrocytic anemia, and low serum folate and red blood cell folate levels.

E. A 25-year-old woman with systemic lupus erythematosus, hemolytic anemia, and positive direct antiglobulin test.

EMQ 3

Match each patient with the most appropriate laboratory test to confirm the diagnosis of their anemia.
1. G6PD enzyme assay.
2. Bone marrow biopsy.
3. Cytogenetic analysis.
4. Hemoglobin electrophoresis.
5. Bone marrow aspiration

A. A 22-year-old woman with thalassemia minor, microcytic hypochromic anemia, and normal serum iron and ferritin levels.
B. A 18-year-old man with glucose-6-phosphate dehydrogenase deficiency, hemolytic anemia, and Heinz bodies on peripheral blood smear.
C. A 27-year-old woman with iron deficiency anemia, microcytic hypochromic anemia, and low serum iron and ferritin levels.
D. A 62-year-old man with myelodysplastic syndrome, macrocytic anemia, and dysplastic cells on peripheral blood smear.
E. A 52-year-old woman with aplastic anemia, pancytopenia, and low reticulocyte count.

EMQ 4

Match each patient with the most appropriate treatment for their anemia.
1. Oral iron supplementation.
2. Hydroxyurea.
3. Intramuscular vitamin B12 injections.
4. Allogeneic stem cell transplantation.
5. Prednisone.

A. A 42-year-old woman with iron deficiency anemia due to menorrhagia.
B. A 37-year-old man with vitamin B12 deficiency anemia due to Crohn's disease.
C. A 28-year-old woman with sickle cell anemia and recurrent pain crises.
D. A 24-year-old man with hemolytic anemia due to warm autoimmune hemolysis.
E. A 19-year-old woman with severe aplastic anemia and matched sibling donor.

EMQ 5

Match each patient with the most likely complication of their anemia.
1. Iron overload
2. Pulmonary infarction.
3. Pigmented gallstones.
4. Esophageal web
5. Subacute combined degeneration of the spinal cord.

A. A 67-year-old man with pernicious anemia and neurological symptoms.
B. A 58-year-old woman with iron deficiency anemia and dysphagia.
C. A 48-year-old man with hemolytic anemia and cholelithiasis.
D. A 38-year-old woman with sickle cell anemia and acute chest syndrome.
E. A 28-year-old man with thalassemia major and hepatomegaly.

EMQ 6

Match each patient with the most likely diagnosis based on their white blood cell count and differential.

1. Leukemoid reaction.
2. Neutropenia.
3. Neutrophilia.
4. Hypersegmented neutrophils.
5. Pelger-Huet anomaly

A. A 25-year-old woman with a history of systemic lupus erythematosus, who presents with fever, sore throat, and fatigue. Her WBC count is 2.1 x 10^9/L, with 60% neutrophils, 30% lymphocytes, 8% monocytes, and 2% eosinophils.

B. A 35-year-old man with a history of Crohn's disease, who is on corticosteroid therapy. His WBC count is 18.5 x 10^9/L, with 80% neutrophils, 15% lymphocytes, 4% monocytes, and 1% eosinophils.

C. A 45-year-old woman with a history of recurrent urinary tract infections, who presents with dysuria, frequency, and flank pain. Her WBC count is 22.3 x 10^9/L, with 88% neutrophils, 8% lymphocytes, 3% monocytes, and 1% eosinophils.

D. A 55-year-old man with a history of alcoholism, who presents with macrocytic anemia and glossitis. His WBC count is 4.8 x 10^9/L, with 40% neutrophils, 50% lymphocytes, 8% monocytes, and 2% eosinophils. His neutrophils have more than five nuclear lobes.

E. A 65-year-old woman with a history of rheumatoid arthritis, who is on methotrexate therapy. Her WBC count is 3.2 x 10^9/L, with 50% neutrophils, 40% lymphocytes, 8% monocytes, and 2% eosinophils. Her neutrophils have two round lobes connected by a thin filament.

EMQ7

Match each patient with the most likely cause of their eosinophilia.

1. Parasitic infection.
2. Hypereosinophilic syndrome.
3. Allergic disorder.
4. Drug reaction.
5. Inflammatory disorder.

A. A 12-year-old boy with a history of asthma and allergic rhinitis, who presents with wheezing, coughing, and nasal congestion. His WBC count is 9.8 x 10^9/L, with 10% eosinophils.

B. A 22-year-old woman with a history of travel to Africa, who presents with abdominal pain, diarrhea, and weight loss. Her stool examination reveals eggs of Schistosoma mansoni. Her WBC count is 11.2 x 10^9/L, with 15% eosinophils.

C. A 32-year-old man with a history of ulcerative colitis, who presents with bloody stools, abdominal cramps, and fever. His WBC count is 12.5 x 10^9/L, with 12% eosinophils.

D. A 42-year-old woman with a history of chronic cough, dyspnea, and skin rash. Her chest X-ray shows bilateral pulmonary infiltrates. Her WBC count is 13.4 x 10^9/L, with 18% eosinophils. Her serum IgE level is elevated.

E. A 52-year-old man with a history of splenomegaly, hepatomegaly, and thrombocytopenia. His bone marrow biopsy shows increased eosinophils and mast cells. His WBC count is 15.6 x 10^9/L, with 20% eosinophils. He has a positive test for FIP1L1-PDGFRA fusion gene.

EMQ 8

Match each patient with the most likely diagnosis based on their lymphocyte morphology.

1. Infectious mononucleosis.
2. Lymphocytosis.
3. Lymphocytopenia.
4. Chronic lymphocytic leukemia.
5. Hairy cell leukemia.

A. A 16-year-old girl with a history of sore throat, fever, and malaise. Her WBC count is 14.2 x 10^9/L, with 60% lymphocytes. Her lymphocytes are large, with abundant cytoplasm and irregular nuclei.

B. A 26-year-old man with a history of HIV infection, who presents with oral candidiasis, diarrhea, and weight loss. His CD4+ T cell count is 150 cells/microliter. His WBC count is 3.8 x 10^9/L, with 20% lymphocytes. His lymphocytes are small, with scanty cytoplasm and round nuclei.

C. A 36-year-old woman with a history of autoimmune hemolytic anemia, who presents with fatigue, pallor, and jaundice. Her WBC count is 12.4 x 10^9/L, with 70% lymphocytes. Her lymphocytes are small to medium, with clumped chromatin and irregular nuclei. Some lymphocytes have projections or villi on their surface.

D. A 46-year-old man with a history of night sweats, weight loss, and lymphadenopathy. His WBC count is 25.6 x 10^9/L, with 80% lymphocytes. His lymphocytes are small, with dense chromatin and indented nuclei. Some lymphocytes have cytoplasmic fragments or projections.

E. A 56-year-old woman with a history of splenomegaly, leukocytosis, and thrombocytosis. Her WBC count is 45.2 x 10^9/L, with 40% lymphocytes. Her lymphocytes are large, with abundant cytoplasm and round or oval nuclei. Some lymphocytes have granules in their cytoplasm.

EMQ 9

Match each patient with the most likely cause of their monocytosis.

1. Chronic myelomonocytic leukemia.
2. Acute monocytic leukemia.
3. Myelodysplastic syndrome.

4. Bacterial infection.
5. Rheumatoid arthritis.

A. A 6-year-old boy with a history of fever, bone pain, and gingival bleeding. His WBC count is 65.4 x 10^9/L, with 40% monocytes. His monocytes are large, with folded nuclei and fine granules. His bone marrow biopsy shows increased blasts with monocytic differentiation.

B. A 66-year-old man with a history of fatigue, weight loss, and splenomegaly. His WBC count is 12.8 x 10^9/L, with 15% monocytes. His monocytes are normal in size and morphology. His bone marrow biopsy shows increased monocytes and dysplasia in erythroid and megakaryocytic lineages.

C. A 76-year-old woman with a history of hypertension, diabetes, and coronary artery disease, who presents with chest pain, dyspnea, and diaphoresis. Her WBC count is 14.2 x 10^9/L, with 12% monocytes. Her monocytes are normal in size and morphology. Her cardiac enzymes are elevated.

D. A 86-year-old man with a history of chronic lymphocytic leukemia, who presents with fever, chills, and night sweats. His WBC count is 98.6 x 10^9/L, with 10% monocytes. His monocytes are normal in size and morphology. His blood culture is positive for Staphylococcus aureus.

E. A 96-year-old woman with a history of osteoarthritis, who presents with joint pain, stiffness, and swelling. Her WBC count is 11.4 x 10^9/L, with 14% monocytes. Her monocytes are normal in size and morphology. Her rheumatoid factor and anti-citrullinated peptide antibodies are positive.

EMQ 10

Match each patient with the most likely type of hematological malignancy based on their clinical presentation and laboratory findings.

1. Acute lymphoblastic leukemia (ALL).
2. Chronic lymphocytic leukemia (CLL).
3. Acute myeloid leukemia (AML).
4. Hodgkin lymphoma.
5. Multiple myeloma.
6. Polycythemia vera.

A. A 65-year-old man with fatigue, weight loss, and night sweats. His CBC shows leukocytosis with 90% lymphocytes, some of which have smudge cells. His flow cytometry shows CD5, CD19, and CD23 positive cells.

B. A 25-year-old woman with fever, bone pain, and gingival bleeding. Her CBC shows pancytopenia with 80% blasts, some of which have Auer rods. Her cytogenetics show t(15;17).

C. A 35-year-old man with pruritus, lymphadenopathy, and splenomegaly. His CBC shows normocytic anemia and eosinophilia. His biopsy shows Reed-Sternberg cells. His immunohistochemistry shows CD15 and CD30 positive cells.

D. A 45-year-old woman with bone pain, renal failure, and hypercalcemia. Her CBC shows normocytic anemia and rouleaux formation. Her serum protein electrophoresis shows a monoclonal spike. Her bone marrow biopsy shows plasma cells.

E. A 55-year-old man with fatigue, splenomegaly, and leukocytosis. His CBC shows increased red blood cells, white blood cells, and platelets. His JAK2 mutation test is positive.

F. A 15-year-old boy with fever, lymphadenopathy, and hepatosplenomegaly. His CBC shows leukocytosis with 85% lymphoblasts. His flow cytometry shows CD10, CD19, and TdT positive cells. His cytogenetics show t(12;21).

EMQ 11

Match each hematological malignancy with the most appropriate treatment option based on the current standard of care.

1. Allogeneic stem cell transplantation.
2. Chemotherapy with cytarabine and anthracycline.
3. Chemotherapy with fludarabine, cyclophosphamide, and rituximab.
4. Chemotherapy with vincristine, prednisone, and asparaginase.
5. Chemotherapy with bortezomib, lenalidomide, and dexamethasone.
6. Phlebotomy and hydroxyurea.

    A. Acute lymphoblastic leukemia (ALL).
    B. Chronic lymphocytic leukemia (CLL).
    C. Acute myeloid leukemia (AML).
    D. Hodgkin lymphoma.
    E. Multiple myeloma.
    F. Polycythemia vera.

EMQ 12

Match each hematological malignancy with the most common cytogenetic or molecular abnormality associated with it.

1. t(9;22) BCR-ABL1.
2. t(15;17) PML-RARA.
3. del(13q) or trisomy 12.
4. t(14;18) BCL2-IGH.
5. t(11;14) CCND1-IGH.
6. EBV infection.

    A. Acute lymphoblastic leukemia (ALL).
    B. Chronic lymphocytic leukemia (CLL).
    C. Acute myeloid leukemia (AML).
    D. Hodgkin lymphoma.
    E. Multiple myeloma.
    F. Mantle cell lymphoma.

EMQ 13

Match each hematological malignancy with the most characteristic immunophenotype based on flow cytometry or immunohistochemistry.

1. CD5, CD19, CD23 positive.
2. CD10, CD19, TdT positive.
3. CD15, CD30 positive.
4. CD34, CD117, MPO positive.
5. CD38, CD138, CD56 positive.
6. CD10, CD19, CD20, BCL2 positive.
    A. Acute lymphoblastic leukemia (ALL).
    B. Chronic lymphocytic leukemia (CLL).
    C. Acute myeloid leukemia (AML).
    D. Hodgkin lymphoma.
    E. Multiple myeloma.
    F. Follicular lymphoma.

EMQ 14

Match each hematological malignancy with the most common complication or adverse outcome associated with it.

1. Tumor lysis syndrome.
2. Richter transformation.
3. Disseminated intravascular coagulation.
4. Secondary malignancies.
5. Amyloidosis.
6. Thrombosis or hemorrhage.
    A. Acute lymphoblastic leukemia (ALL).
    B. Chronic lymphocytic leukemia (CLL).
    C. Acute myeloid leukemia (AML).
    D. Hodgkin lymphoma.
    E. Multiple myeloma.
    F. Polycythemia vera.

EMQ 15

Match each patient with the most likely type of polycythemia based on their clinical presentation and laboratory findings.

1. Primary polycythemia.
2. Secondary polycythemia.
3. Relative polycythemia.
    A. A 32-year-old woman who lives in a high-altitude area and has a history of chronic smoking. She presents with headache, dizziness, and fatigue. Her hemoglobin is 18.5 g/dL and her hematocrit is 55%. Her serum erythropoietin level is normal.
    B. A 42-year-old man who has a history of chronic obstructive pulmonary disease. He presents with dyspnea, cyanosis, and clubbing. His hemoglobin is 19.2 g/dL and his hematocrit is 57%. His serum erythropoietin level is elevated.
    C. A 52-year-old woman who has a history of hypertension and diabetes. She presents with pruritus, abdominal pain, and splenomegaly. Her hemoglobin is 20.4 g/dL and her hematocrit is

60%. Her serum erythropoietin level is low. She has a positive test for JAK2 mutation.

EMQ 16

Match each patient with the most appropriate treatment for their polycythemia.

1. Phlebotomy.
2. Hydroxyurea.
3. Surgery.
4. Fluid replacement.
5. Ruxolitinib.

A. A 62-year-old woman who has polycythemia vera and a history of recurrent thrombosis. She presents with chest pain and shortness of breath. Her hemoglobin is 21.6 g/dL and her hematocrit is 64%. She has a positive test for JAK2 mutation.

B. A 72-year-old man who has secondary polycythemia due to renal cell carcinoma. He presents with hematuria, flank pain, and weight loss. His hemoglobin is 18.8 g/dL and his hematocrit is 56%. His serum erythropoietin level is elevated.

C. A 82-year-old woman who has relative polycythemia due to dehydration. She presents with confusion, dry mouth, and constipation. Her hemoglobin is 17.2 g/dL and her hematocrit is 52%. Her serum erythropoietin level is normal.

D. A 92-year-old man who has polycythemia vera and a history of peptic ulcer disease. He presents with melena, anemia, and iron deficiency. His hemoglobin is 16.4 g/dL and his hematocrit is 49%. He has a positive test for JAK2 mutation.

E. A 22-year-old woman who has secondary polycythemia due to congenital heart disease. She presents with cyanosis, clubbing, and palpitations. Her hemoglobin is 19.6 g/dL and her hematocrit is 58%. Her serum erythropoietin level is elevated.

EMQ 17

Match each patient with the most likely complication of their polycythemia.

1. Gout.
2. Stroke.
3. Pulmonary embolism.
4. Myelofibrosis.
5. Aquagenic pruritus.

A. A 44-year-old woman who has polycythemia vera and a history of migraine. She presents with visual disturbances, weakness, and slurred speech. Her hemoglobin is 20.8 g/dL and her hematocrit is 62%. She has a positive test for JAK2 mutation.

B. A 54-year-old man who has secondary polycythemia due to sleep apnea. He presents with snoring, daytime sleepiness, and hypertension. His hemoglobin is 18.4 g/dL and his hematocrit is 55%. His serum erythropoietin level is elevated.

C. A 64-year-old woman who has polycythemia vera and a history of pruritus. She presents with itching, especially after a hot shower. Her hemoglobin is 19.2 g/dL and her hematocrit is 57%. She has a positive test for JAK2 mutation.

D. A 74-year-old man who has polycythemia vera and a history of gout. He presents with joint pain, swelling, and redness. His hemoglobin is 21.6 g/dL and his hematocrit is 64%. He has a positive test for JAK2 mutation.

E. A 84-year-old woman who has polycythemia vera and a history of splenomegaly. She presents with abdominal discomfort, early satiety, and weight loss. Her hemoglobin is 20.4 g/dL and her hematocrit is 61%. She has a positive test for JAK2 mutation.

EMQ 18

Match each patient with the most appropriate laboratory test to confirm the diagnosis of their polycythemia.

1. Arterial blood gas.
2. Carboxyhemoglobin.
3. Chest X-ray.
4. Bone marrow biopsy.
5. Abdominal ultrasound.

A. A 26-year-old man who has a history of living in a high-altitude area. He presents with headache, dizziness, and fatigue. His hemoglobin is 18.5 g/dL and his hematocrit is 55%. His serum erythropoietin level is normal.

B. A 36-year-old woman who has a history of chronic smoking. She presents with dyspnea, cyanosis, and clubbing. Her hemoglobin is 19.2 g/dL and her hematocrit is 57%. Her serum erythropoietin level is elevated.

C. A 46-year-old man who has a history of chronic obstructive pulmonary disease. He presents with cough, sputum, and wheezes. His hemoglobin is 20.4 g/dL and his hematocrit is 60%. His serum erythropoietin level is low. He has a positive test for JAK2 mutation.

D. A 56-year-old woman who has a history of hypertension and diabetes. She presents with pruritus, abdominal pain, and splenomegaly. Her hemoglobin is 21.6 g/dL and her hematocrit is 64%. Her serum erythropoietin level is low. She has a positive test for JAK2 mutation.

E. A 66-year-old man who has a history of renal cell carcinoma. He presents with hematuria, flank pain, and weight loss. His hemoglobin is 18.8 g/dL and his hematocrit is 56%. His serum erythropoietin level is elevated.

EMQ 19

Match each patient with the most appropriate preventive measure to reduce the risk of thrombotic complications of their polycythemia.

1. Aspirin.

2. Continuous positive airway pressure.
3. Low molecular weight heparin.
4. Phlebotomy.
5. Fluid intake.

A. A 34-year-old woman who has polycythemia vera and a history of recurrent miscarriages. She presents with amenorrhea and a positive pregnancy test. Her hemoglobin is 19.6 g/dL and her hematocrit is 58%. She has a positive test for JAK2 mutation.

B. A 44-year-old man who has secondary polycythemia due to sleep apnea. He presents with snoring, daytime sleepiness, and hypertension. His hemoglobin is 18.4 g/dL and his hematocrit is 55%. His serum erythropoietin level is elevated.

C. A 54-year-old woman who has polycythemia vera and a history of deep vein thrombosis. She presents with leg swelling, pain, and redness. Her hemoglobin is 20.8 g/dL and her hematocrit is 62%. She has a positive test for JAK2 mutation.

D. A 64-year-old man who has polycythemia vera and a history of angina. He presents with chest pain and shortness of breath. His hemoglobin is 21.6 g/dL and his hematocrit is 64%. He has a positive test for JAK2 mutation.

E. A 74-year-old woman who has relative polycythemia due to dehydration. She presents with confusion, dry mouth, and constipation. Her hemoglobin is 17.2 g/dL and her hematocrit is 52%. Her serum erythropoietin level is normal.

EMQ 20

For each case description, select the appropriate category of acute leukemia.

A. Acute lymphoblastic leukemia (ALL) - B-cell
B. Acute lymphoblastic leukemia (ALL) - T-cell
C. Acute myeloid leukemia (AML) with favorable risk
D. Acute myeloid leukemia (AML) with intermediate risk
E. Acute myeloid leukemia (AML) with unfavorable risk
F. Acute promyelocytic leukemia (APL)
G. Blastic plasmacytoid dendritic cell neoplasm (BPDCN)

1. A 25-year-old man presents with fatigue, pallor, and lymphadenopathy. Laboratory findings reveal pancytopenia, and peripheral blood film displays lymphoblasts. Immunophenotyping confirms the presence of T-cell lymphoblasts expressing CD3, CD4, and CD8.

2. A 60-year-old woman is diagnosed with leukemia following complaints of fatigue, bruising, and weight loss. Peripheral blood film demonstrates myeloblasts without maturation beyond the myeloblast stage. Cytogenetic analysis reveals inv(16)(p13.1q22) or t(16;16)(p13.1;q22).

3. A 45-year-old man is found to have leukopenia, anemia, and

thrombocytopenia. Blood film reveals myeloid blasts expressing CD13, CD33, and CD117. Complex karyotype alterations are identified.

4. A 30-year-old woman is diagnosed with acute leukemia displaying promyelocytes with abundant azurophilic granules and Auer rods on blood film. Cytogenetic analysis reveals t(15;17)(q22;q12).

5. G: A 55-year-old man presents with extensive cutaneous involvement, marked by violaceous patches and nodules. Biopsy reveals a monomorphic infiltrate composed of medium-sized blast cells with round nuclei, finely dispersed chromatin, and indistinct nucleoli. Immunostain highlights positivity for CD4, CD56, and CD123.

EMQ 21

Match the case descriptions to the recommended initial therapies.

A. Induction chemotherapy followed by consolidation chemo-radiotherapy

B. Combination of daunorubicin, cytarabine, and etoposide

C. High-dose cytarabine plus mitoxantrone

D. Standard induction chemotherapy

E. Tyrosine kinase inhibitor (TKI) and all-trans retinoic acid (ATRA)

F. Hyperfractionated cyclophosphamide, vincristine, doxorubicin, and dexamethasone (hyperCVAD) alternating with high-dose methotrexate and cytarabine

G. Autologous stem cell transplantation

    1. A 20-year-old female with Burkitt leukemia

    2. A 50-year-old male with AML harboring FLT3 internal tandem duplication

    3. A 30-year-old female with newly diagnosed APL

    4. A 65-year-old male with newly diagnosed DLBCL involving bone marrow

    5. A 40-year-old female with Ph-negative ALL having good risk characteristics.

EMQ 22

Select the suitable measure for addressing the given issues.

A. Administration of colony-stimulating factors

B. Strict infection control measures

C. Leukopheresis

D. Red cell transfusion

E. Platelet transfusion

F. Management of tumor lysis syndrome

G. Nutrition counseling

    1. Preventing infectious complications in neutropenic patients

    2. Managing life-threatening bleeding in a patient with profound thrombocytopenia

    3. Addressing severe anemia in a patient with acute leukemia

    4. Removing excess white blood cells to decrease the risk of tumor lysis syndrome

5. Encouraging adequate nutrition intake and preventing cachexia in patients undergoing treatment

EMQ 23

Identify the possible complications associated with the listed situations.
A. Differentiation syndrome
B. Cardiac tamponade
C. Posterior reversible encephalopathy syndrome (PRES)
D. Invasion of the epidural space
E. Tumor lysis syndrome
F. Superior vena cava syndrome
G. Sweet's syndrome

1. Development of a painful, tender, warm, erythematous patch with surrounding edema in a patient with AML treated with ATRA
2. Sudden onset of severe headache, altered mental status, visual disturbances, and seizures in a patient with acute leukemia
3. Rapid reduction in urinary output, hyperkalemia, hyperphosphatemia, and hypocalcemia in a patient with acute leukemia initiating intensive chemotherapy
4. Progressive shortness of breath, stridor, and facial plethora in a patient with acute leukemia
5. New-onset pericardial friction rub, jugular venous distention, and Beck's triad in a patient with acute leukemia

EMQ 24

Determine the long-term sequelae or late effect linked to the described treatments.
A. Avascular necrosis
B. Growth hormone deficiency
C. Pulmonary fibrosis
D. Gonadal dysfunction
E. Increased risk of secondary malignancies
F. Learning disabilities
G. Persistent sinus bradycardia

1. Craniospinal radiotherapy in a 10-year-old child with medulloblastoma
2. Total body irradiation prior to autologous stem cell transplantation
3. Maintenance chemotherapy consisting of mercaptopurine and methotrexate for a patient with ALL
4. High cumulative doses of anthracyclines in a patient with AML
5. Busulfan and cyclophosphamide conditioning regimen before allogeneic stem cell transplantation

EMQ 25

Match the clinical features with the appropriate chronic leukemia type.
A. Chronic myeloid leukemia (CML)
B. Chronic lymphocytic leukemia (CLL)/small lymphocytic lymphoma (SLL)
C. Prolymphocytic leukemia (PLL)

D. Hair follicle center lymphoma (HFCL)

E. Large granular lymphocytic leukemia (LGLL)

F. Sezary syndrome (SS)

G. Follicular lymphoma (FL)

    1. Predominantly affects elderly individuals

    2. Presents with massive splenomegaly

    3. Often accompanied by peripheral lymphadenopathy

    4. Associated with skin lesions and pruritis

    5. Can arise from hair follicles

    6. Typically manifests as a progressive increase in absolute neutrophil count

    7. Occurs predominately in middle-aged to older adults

EMQ 26

Associate the molecular genetics with the corresponding chronic leukemia.

A. Philadelphia chromosome (Ph)

B. t(11;14)(q13;q32)

C. t(8;14)(q24;q32)

D. Trisomy 12

E. RUNX1/ETO fusion

F. ATM mutation

G. BCOR mutation

    1. Constitutively active tyrosine kinase resulting in uncontrolled proliferation

    2. Overexpression of cyclin D1 promoting entry into the cell cycle

    3. Formation of MYC-IGH fusion protein driving lymphocyte transformation

    4. Mutation commonly observed in CLL/SLL, particularly in familial cases

    5. Aberrant expression of runt-related transcription factor 1

    6. Triplicated allele seen in approximately 15–20% of CLL cases

    7. Somatic mutation occurring in around half of CLL/SLL patients

EMQ 27

Select the proper diagnostic method for identifying each chronic leukemia.

A. Conventional cytogenetics

B. Fluorescence in situ hybridization (FISH)

C. Next-generation sequencing (NGS)

D. Immunophenotyping by flow cytometry

E. Histopathological examination of excised lymph node

F. BCR: ABL1 quantitative PCR assay

G. Southern blot analysis

    1. Detecting submicroscopic deletions in del(17p) or del(11q)

    2. Identifying reciprocal translocation between chromosomes 9 and 22

    3. Quantitating BCR: ABL1 transcripts

    4. Assessing the clonal expansion of lymphocytes

    5. Screening for the presence of the Philadelphia chromosome

6. Determining the somatic mutations present in leukemic cells

EMQ 28

Select the appropriate frontline treatment option for each chronic leukemia type.

A. Interferon-α

B. Imatinib

C. Alemtuzumab

D. Bruton's tyrosine kinase (BTK) inhibitor

E. Cyclophosphamide, vincristine, and prednisone (CVP)

F. Watch and wait

G. Radioimmunotherapy (RIT)

1. Frontline management for asymptomatic, stable-phase CML

2. Treatment for newly diagnosed mantle cell lymphoma

3. Initial therapy for previously untreated CLL/SLL

4. Optimal treatment for young, fit patients with advanced-stage FL

5. Standard of care for CD52-positive CLL/SLL

EMQ 29

Identify the indicated targeted therapy for each chronic leukemia type.

A. Dasatinib

B. Bosutinib

C. Ibrutinib

D. Venetoclax

E. Ponatinib

F. Lenalidomide

G. Obinutuzumab

1. Treatment for CML refractory to imatinib

2. Treatment for CLL/SLL with del(17p)

3. Monotherapy for CLL/SLL carrying TP53 or SF3B1 mutations

4. Targeted agent approved for both CLL/SLL and mantle cell lymphoma

5. Agent combined with rituximab for treating FL

EMQ 30

Identify the underlying cause of secondary polycythemia for each given scenario.

A. Smoking

B. Sleep apnea

C. Living at altitude

D. Renal artery stenosis

E. Androgen abuse

F. Polycythemia due to carbon monoxide exposure

G. Familial erythrocytosis

1. A 60-year-old male lifelong smoker presenting with plethoric facies and erythrocytosis

2. A 45-year-old obese male experiencing sleep apnea and concomitant erythrocytosis

3. A 35-year-old resident living near sea level complaining of fatigue, dyspnea, and erythrocytosis
4. A 50-year-old female suffering from renovascular hypertension caused by renal artery stenosis and accompanying erythrocytosis
5. A 70-year-old male taking testosterone replacement therapy and developing erythrocytosis

EMQ 31

Assign the appropriate multiple myeloma presentation to each case description.

A. Hyperproteinemia and hyperviscosity.
B. Pathologic fracture
C. Normocytic anemia
D. Castleman disease
E. Spontaneous bleeding
F. Infection
G. Kidney dysfunction

    1. A 65-year-old male with weakness, dyspnea, and dark urine
    2. A 70-year-old female suffering from sudden bone pain and collapse
    3. A 55-year-old male with recurrent upper respiratory tract infections
    4. A 60-year-old female with decreasing estimated glomerular filtration rate (eGFR)
    5. A 75-year-old male with spontaneous bleeds and petechiae

EMQ 32

Classify each multiple myeloma case based on the revised International Staging System (ISS-R).

A. Stage I
B. Stage II
C. Stage III

    1. A 60-year-old male with albumin 4.5 g/dL, beta-2 microglobulin 2.5 mg/L, and normal lactic dehydrogenase (LDH)
    2. A 55-year-old female with albumin 3.2 g/dL, beta-2 microglobulin 4.0 mg/L, and normal LDH
    3. A 65-year-old male with albumin 2.8 g/dL, beta-2 microglobulin 6.0 mg/L, and elevated LDH

EMQ 33

Select the primary objective for managing multiple myeloma in each case.

A. Best supportive care
B. Deep response aimed at achieving stringent complete response (sCR)
C. Slow disease progression

    1. A 60-year-old otherwise healthy female seeking aggressive treatment
    2. An 80-year-old male with significant comorbidities and limited functional ability
    3. A 75-year-old male with slow-progressing multiple myeloma

EMQ 34

Match the consequence with the corresponding causative mechanism.
A. Hypercalcemia
B. Ammonia toxicity
C. Spinal cord compression
D. Anemia
E. Renal failure
F. Hyperviscosity syndrome
G. Recurrent infections
    1. Destruction of bone matrix releasing calcium
    2. Accumulation of light chains in the tubular lumina
    3. Impairment of humoral and cell-mediated immunity
    4. Suppression of erythropoiesis due to bone marrow invasion
    5. Elevation of Bence Jones protein hindering renal clearance
    6. Crowded vessels reducing blood flow velocity
    7. Production of ammonia by urea-splitting bacteria

EMQ 35

Match the characteristics with the corresponding lymphoma subtype.
A. Hodgkin lymphoma
B. Diffuse large B-cell lymphoma
C. Follicular lymphoma
D. Marginal zone lymphoma
E. Mantle cell lymphoma
F. Small lymphocytic lymphoma
G. Classic Hodgkin lymphoma
    1. Reed-Sternberg cells
    2. Germinal centers containing centroblasts and centrocytes
    3. Most common primary extranodal site being the ocular adnexae
    4. Usually low grade with an indolent course
    5. Associated with the characteristic t(11;14)(q13;q32) translocation

EMQ 36

Classify the stages of Hodgkin lymphoma utilizing the modified Ann Arbor Staging System.
A. Stage I
B. Stage II
C. Stage III
D. Stage IV
    1. Two or more lymph node regions on the same side of the diaphragm involved
    2. Single lymph node region or single extra-nodal organ affected
    3. Diffuse involvement of one or more organs outside the lymphatic system
    4. Lymph node regions on both sides of the diaphragm involved

EMQ 37

Match the immunohistochemistry marker with the corresponding lymphoma subset.

A. PAX5

B. CD10

C. CD20

D. CD3

E. ALK

F. CD30

G. CD138

    1. B-cell lymphomas

    2. T-cell lymphomas

    3. Hodgkin lymphoma

    4. Anaplastic large cell lymphoma

    5. Multiple myeloma

EMQ 38

Match each type of lymphoma with the most common gene mutation associated with it. Choose the best answer from the list of options.

A. CCND1

B. TP53

C. MYD88

D. BCL2

E. BCL6

    1. Mantle cell lymphoma

    2. Diffuse large B-cell lymphoma

    3. Follicular lymphoma

    4. Burkitt lymphoma

    5. Waldenström macroglobulinemia

EMQ 39

Assign the platelet function disorder to the corresponding description.

A. Storage pool deficiency

B. Congenital afibrinogenemia

C. Von Willebrand disease

D. Bernard-Soulier syndrome

E. Glanzmann thrombasthenia

F. Gray platelet syndrome

G. Scott syndrome

    1. Qualitative platelet disorder with decreased surface integrin $\alpha IIb\beta 3$

    2. Disorder characterized by giant platelets and impaired platelet aggregation

    3. Platelets exhibit reduced dense granule release and diminished platelet activation

    4. Congenital absence of von Willebrand factor leads to impaired platelet adhesion

5. Surface integrin αIIbβ3 is completely missing, resulting in severe bleeding tendencies

6. Platelets possess reduced amounts of dense and alpha granules

EMQ 40

Match the diagnostic tools with the corresponding platelet disorder investigation.

A. aggregometry

B. Electron microscopy

C. Flow cytometry

D. Thrombelastogram

E. Bleeding time Light transmission

F. Activated partial thromboplastin time

G. Prothrombin time

1. Testing platelet aggregation patterns in response to specific agents
2. Visualizing ultrastructure of platelets to identify structural anomalies
3. Monitoring global clot formation dynamics in vitro
4. Enumerating platelet surface markers to assess platelet functionality
5. Estimating susceptibility to bleeding by evaluating capillary perfusion

EMQ 41

Select the appropriate intervention for the outlined platelet function disorder.

A. Fresh frozen plasma

B. Desmopressin (DDAVP)

C. Corticosteroids

D. Recombinant factor VIIa

E. Platelet transfusion

F. Antifibrinolytics

G. Hormonal contraception

1. Afibrinogenemia
2. Type 1 von Willebrand disease
3. Menorrhagia induced by platelet function disorder
4. Severe bleeding episode in a patient with Glanzmann thrombasthenia
5. Preoperative preparation for a patient with platelet storage pool deficiency

EMQ 42

Assign the coagulation disorder to the corresponding description.

A. Hemophilia A

B. Hemophilia B

C. Vitamin K deficiency

D. Liver disease

E. Warfarin therapy

F. Factor XII deficiency

G. Dysfibrinogenemia

1. Coagulation disorder with a deficiency in factor VIII

2. Condition with reduced factor IX levels
3. Insufficient production of functional coagulation factors due to impaired liver synthetic capability
4. Syndrome caused by insufficient vitamin K availability
5. Inhibition of vitamin K-dependent coagulation factors due to warfarin ingestion
6. Diminished or dysfunctional fibrinogen molecules
7. Deficiency of contact phase coagulation protein

EMQ 43

Match the diagnostic techniques with the corresponding coagulation disorder investigations.

A. Prothrombin time (PT)
B. Activated partial thromboplastin time (aPTT)
C. Mixing study
D. Thrombin time (TT)
E. Fibrinogen assay
F. Specific coagulation factor assays
G. Platelet count

    1. Assessment of factor VIII activity
    2. Analysis of contact phase coagulation proteins
    3. Global screening test for intrinsic and final common pathways
    4. Overall measurement of the conversion of fibrinogen to fibrin
    5. Evaluation of overall hemostatic capability including platelets and the extrinsic and common pathways
    6. Investigation of specific factor activities

EMQ 44

Select the appropriate interventions for the outlined coagulation disorders.

A. Fresh frozen plasma
B. Purified coagulation factor concentrates
C. Vitamin K supplementation
D. Prothrombin complex concentrate
E. Fibrinogen supplementation
F. Desmopressin (DDAVP)
G. Oral anticoagulation withdrawal

    1. Moderate to severe factor VIII deficiency
    2. Factor IX deficiency
    3. Mild to moderate factor deficiency with planned invasive procedure
    4. Disseminated intravascular coagulation (DIC)
    5. Excessive anticoagulation due to oral anticoagulant therapy
    6. Heparin-induced thrombocytopenia (HIT)

EMQ 45

Assign the appropriate blood component to the corresponding clinical indication.

A. Packed red blood cells
B. Whole blood
C. Fresh frozen plasma
D. Platelets
E. Cryoprecipitate
F. Albumin
G. Granulocytes

1. Restoration of intravascular volume
2. Correction of hypovolemic shock
3. Compensation for severe anemia
4. Providing clotting factors
5. Administering platelets
6. Augmenting fibrinogen levels
7. Infusing colloids for maintaining oncotic pressure

EMQ 46

Link the labeling requirement to its corresponding rationale.

A. Unit identification number
B. Donor identification number
C. Collection date
D. ABO group
E. Rh type
F. Expiration date
G. Blood bank inventory location code

1. Required for tracking purposes during recall events
2. Helps prevent clerical errors
3. Facilitates determination of remaining shelf life
4. Crucial for ensuring compatibility during transfusion
5. Important for providing type-specific products to Rh-negative females
6. Critical in selecting appropriate units for specific patients
7. Useful for efficient allocation and retrieval of blood products

EMQ 47

Select the correct crossmatch technique for each situation.

A. Major crossmatch
B. Minor crossmatch
C. Simultaneous minor crossmatch
D. Automated computerized crossmatch
E. Bedside emergency crossmatch

1. Before issuing blood to a new patient with unknown antibody screen results
2. Prior to transfusing a repeat patient whose last antibody screen showed no clinically significant antibodies

3. When immediate transfusion is necessary, and the automated crossmatch is delayed or unavailable
4. In urgent situations where rapid antibody detection is crucial
5. Utilizing electronic data systems for routine, elective procedures

EMQ 48

Match the risks associated with blood transfusion to their consequences.

A. Transmission of infectious diseases
B. Hemolytic reactions
C. Metabolic derangements
D. Transfusion-related acute lung injury (TRALI)
E. Transfusion-associated circulatory overload (TACO)
F. Immune suppression
G. Allergic reactions

    1. Delayed recovery from illness or operation
    2. Respiratory distress and fluid accumulation
    3. Acute renal failure
    4. Shortened survival of transfused red blood cells
    5. Life-threatening cardiopulmonary compromise
    6. Bronchospasm, hives, or angioedema
    7. Possibility of acquiring fatal or debilitating infections

EMQ 49

Match the alternative solution with the conventional blood product counterpart.

A. Artificial oxygen carriers
B. Recombinant activated factor VII (rFVIIa)
C. Heat-treated platelets
D. Autologous blood salvage devices
E. Blood substitutes
F. Erythropoietin analogs
G. Photopheresis

    1. Red blood cell substitute
    2. Fibrin sealant
    3. Apheresis-derived platelets processed to reduce bacterial burden
    4. Devices collecting shed blood during surgical procedures for later infusion
    5. Alternative to traditional plasma derivatives
    6. Endogenous stimulator of erythropoiesis
    7. White blood cell removal technology

EMQ 50

Select the appropriate component ratios for managing massive transfusion scenarios.

A. 1:1:1
B. 1:1:2
C. 2:1:1

D. 1:2:1

E. 1:2:2

F. 1:1:4

G. 1:3:1

1. Trauma patients requiring resuscitation with balanced ratios
2. Cardiovascular surgeries necessitating high-volume support
3. Orthopedic operations demanding substantial input
4. Jehovah's Witnesses rejecting transfusion yet needing surgical intervention
5. Pediatric patients undergoing extensive procedures

Section 4:
Single Best Answers, Answers to Questions 1-125

SBA 1: c) Bone marrow
In adults, erythropoiesis primarily occurs in the bone marrow, particularly in the pelvis, sternum, and ribs.
SBA 2: b) Erythropoietin
Erythropoietin, a hormone produced mainly by the kidneys, stimulates the production of red blood cells in the bone marrow.
SBA 3: b) Low oxygen levels
The release of erythropoietin is triggered by hypoxia or low oxygen levels in the blood, signaling the need for more red blood cells to enhance oxygen transport.
SBA 4: c) Vitamin B12
Vitamin B12 is crucial for DNA synthesis in rapidly dividing cells, including erythroblasts in the bone marrow during erythropoiesis.
SBA 5: c) Proerythroblast
The proerythroblast is the earliest committed cell in the erythroid lineage and marks the beginning of erythropoiesis.
SBA 6: b) Iron
Iron is a critical component of hemoglobin, the oxygen-carrying protein in red blood cells, and is essential for its synthesis during erythropoiesis.
SBA 7: c) It increases red blood cell production.
 Erythropoietin stimulates the bone marrow to increase the production of red blood cells, a process known as erythropoiesis.
SBA 8: d) Orthochromatophilic erythroblast
The orthochromatophilic erythroblast, also known as normoblast, is the last nucleated stage in erythropoiesis before the nucleus is expelled to form a reticulocyte.
SBA 9: b) Decrease in cytoplasmic volume.
As erythroid precursors mature, there is a reduction in both cell size and cytoplasmic volume, with an increase in hemoglobin concentration.
SBA 10: c) They undergo apoptosis.
Erythroblasts that fail to synthesize enough hemoglobin are typically removed by apoptosis, a programmed cell death process, to maintain erythrocyte quality.
SBA 11: b) Chronic blood loss
Chronic blood loss, often from the gastrointestinal tract, is a common cause of anemia in the elderly, leading to iron deficiency.
SBA 12: d) Hemolytic anemia
The combination of anemia, jaundice, and an elevated reticulocyte count suggests increased red blood cell destruction, consistent with hemolytic anemia.
SBA13: b) Decreased serum ferritin
Decreased serum ferritin is indicative of depleted iron stores and is a key laboratory finding in iron deficiency anemia.
SBA 14: d) Iron deficiency anemia

Iron deficiency anemia is the most common type of anemia globally, often due to poor diet, blood loss, or increased need for iron such as during pregnancy.

SBA 15: c) Vitamin B12

Vitamin B12 deficiency can lead to megaloblastic anemia, characterized by the presence of large, immature red blood cells due to impaired DNA synthesis.

SBA 16: d) Sickle cells

In sickle cell anemia, red blood cells take on a characteristic crescent or "sickle" shape due to abnormal hemoglobin that causes cells to become rigid and sticky.

SBA 17: d) Chronic kidney disease

Chronic kidney disease is not a direct cause of hemolytic anemia. Hemolytic anemia is caused by the premature destruction of red blood cells, which can be due to autoimmune disorders, genetic defects, infectious agents, or certain medications.

SBA 18: b) Regular blood transfusions

The main treatment for thalassemia major, a severe form of thalassemia, is regular blood transfusions to maintain adequate hemoglobin levels and suppress ineffective erythropoiesis.

SBA 19: d) Low serum iron

Iron deficiency anemia is characterized by low serum iron levels, low serum ferritin, high TIBC, low MCV (microcytic anemia), and a low reticulocyte count.

SBA 20: c) Chronic inflammation

Anemia of chronic disease, also known as anemia of inflammation, is primarily caused by chronic inflammation, which affects iron metabolism and erythropoiesis.

SBA 21: e) Elevated serum iron

Pernicious anemia is associated with vitamin B12 deficiency due to autoimmune gastritis leading to impaired absorption of vitamin B12. It does not typically cause elevated serum iron levels.

SBA 22: b) Autosomal dominant

Hereditary spherocytosis is most commonly inherited in an autosomal dominant pattern, characterized by the presence of spherocytes in the blood due to a defect in red blood cell membrane proteins.

SBA 23: c) Fatigue

Fatigue is a common symptom of anemia due to the reduced oxygen-carrying capacity of the blood, leading to decreased oxygen delivery to tissues.

SBA 24: c) Bone marrow failure

Aplastic anemia is characterized by bone marrow failure, resulting in pancytopenia, which includes a reduction in red blood cells, white blood cells, and platelets.

SBA 25: d) Elevated indirect bilirubin
Hemolytic anemia typically presents with elevated indirect bilirubin due to
the breakdown of red blood cells, along with low haptoglobin, high LDH,
and increased reticulocyte count..
SBA 26: c) It inhibits erythropoiesis.
Lead poisoning inhibits erythropoiesis by interfering with several enzymes
involved in the heme synthesis pathway, leading to anemia.
SBA 27: b) Vitamin B12 deficiency
Vitamin B12 deficiency can lead to macrocytic anemia, characterized by
large red blood cells due to impaired DNA synthesis.
SBA 28: b) Iron deficiency
Iron deficiency is the most common cause of anemia in pregnancy due to
increased iron requirements for the growing fetus and placenta, as well as
blood volume expansion.
SBA 29: d) High reticulocyte count
Fanconi anemia is characterized by bone marrow failure, increased risk of
malignancies, macrocytosis, and congenital abnormalities. It does not
typically present with a high reticulocyte count.
SBA 30: d) Detecting antibodies against red blood cells
The Coombs test, also known as the antiglobulin test, is used to detect
antibodies that are bound to the surface of red blood cells, commonly used
in the diagnosis of autoimmune hemolytic anemias.
SBA 31: b) Chronic renal failure
Chronic renal failure can lead to normocytic anemia due to decreased
production of erythropoietin, which is necessary for red blood cell
production.
SBA 32: d) Thrombocytopenia
Infectious mononucleosis typically presents with fever, pharyngitis,
splenomegaly, and atypical lymphocytes. Thrombocytopenia is not a
characteristic feature.
SBA 33: b) Bacterial infections
Neutrophilia, an increase in neutrophil count, is most commonly caused by
bacterial infections.
SBA 34
SBA 34: a) Eosinophilia
Eosinophilia is defined as an absolute increase in the number of eosinophils
in the blood.
SBA 35: d) All of the above
Leukocytosis, an increase in white blood cell count, can be a physiological
response to stressors such as sleep, exercise, and eating.
SBA 36: c) Large granular lymphocytic leukemia
Large granular lymphocytic leukemia is a benign disorder characterized by
the clonal proliferation of large granular lymphocytes.

SBA 37: b) Hyposegmented neutrophils
Pelger-Huët anomaly is a benign inherited condition characterized by hyposegmented neutrophils.
SBA 38: b) Monocytosis
Monocytosis is characterized by an increased number of circulating monocytes and can be a response to chronic inflammation or infection.
SBA 39: b) Viral infections
In children, lymphocytosis, an increase in lymphocyte count, is typically caused by viral infections.
SBA 40: d) High neutrophil count
CLL is characterized by an increased number of lymphocytes, not neutrophils. It also presents with lymphadenopathy, splenomegaly, increased risk of infections, and smudge cells on peripheral blood smear.
SBA 41: d) All of the above
Reactive lymphocytosis can occur due to various stressors, including smoking, psychological stress, and physical exercise. It is a transient increase in lymphocyte count in response to these factors.
SBA 42: c) Phagocytosis
Platelets are primarily involved in hemostasis and do not perform phagocytosis, which is a function of white blood cells.
SBA 43: c) Von Willebrand disease
Von Willebrand disease is the most common inherited bleeding disorder and is caused by a deficiency of von Willebrand factor, which helps platelets to stick to the blood vessel wall and to each other.
SBA 44: a) Factor VIII
Hemophilia A is caused by a deficiency of Factor VIII, which is essential for the intrinsic pathway of the coagulation cascade.
SBA 45: c) Corticosteroids
The initial treatment for acute ITP typically involves corticosteroids to reduce platelet destruction by the immune system.
SBA 46: c) Activated partial thromboplastin time (aPTT)
Hemophilia A affects the intrinsic pathway of the coagulation cascade, which is assessed by the aPTT test.
SBA 47: b) Prolonged PT and aPTT
DIC is characterized by widespread activation of the coagulation system, leading to prolonged PT and aPTT, low fibrinogen levels, increased D-dimer, and thrombocytopenia.
SBA 48: c) Drug-induced thrombocytopenia
Drug-induced thrombocytopenia is an acquired condition where certain medications can cause a decrease in platelet count.
SBA 49: d) Primary hemostasis
Von Willebrand disease affects primary hemostasis by impairing platelet adhesion to the site of vascular injury.
SBA 50: c) Bypassing agents like recombinant Factor VIIa

In patients with Hemophilia A and inhibitors to Factor VIII, bypassing agents like recombinant Factor VIIa are used to circumvent the inhibited coagulation factor.

SBA 51: e) Elevated prothrombin time (PT)

TTP does not typically cause an elevated PT. It is characterized by fever, microangiopathic hemolytic anemia, neurological symptoms, renal impairment, and thrombocytopenia.

SBA 52: b) Vitamin K deficiency

Vitamin K deficiency is the most common cause of acquired coagulation factor deficiency, affecting factors II, VII, IX, and X.

SBA 53: a) Deficiency of GPIIb/IIIa receptors on platelets

Glanzmann thrombasthenia is a rare genetic platelet disorder characterized by a deficiency of GPIIb/IIIa receptors, leading to impaired platelet aggregation.

SBA 54: d) Factor X

Factor X, also known as the Stuart-Prower factor, is involved in both the intrinsic and extrinsic pathways and is essential for the conversion of prothrombin to thrombin.

SBA 55: b) Desmopressin (DDAVP)

Desmopressin (DDAVP) is the mainstay of treatment for von Willebrand disease as it increases the release of von Willebrand factor from endothelial cells.

SBA 56: a) Prolonged antibiotic therapy

Prolonged antibiotic therapy can lead to Vitamin K deficiency by disrupting the gut flora that synthesizes vitamin K.

SBA 57: c) Factor VIII

In liver disease, Factor VIII levels are typically not decreased and may even be elevated due to increased synthesis by endothelial cells.

SBA 58: b) Activation of antithrombin III

Heparin primarily works by activating antithrombin III, which then inhibits thrombin and Factor Xa.

SBA 59: c) Prolonged bleeding time

Hemophilia B does not typically cause a prolonged bleeding time, which is a measure of platelet function. Hemophilia B affects the intrinsic pathway of the coagulation.

SBA 60: d) Rivaroxaban

Rivaroxaban is a direct oral anticoagulant that selectively inhibits Factor Xa, preventing thrombin generation and thrombus formation.

SBA 61: c) Spontaneous bleeding

A platelet count of 20,000/μL is significantly below the normal range, putting the patient at risk for spontaneous bleeding due to insufficient platelet-mediated hemostasis.

SBA 62: c) Discontinue heparin and start a non-heparin anticoagulant

The primary treatment for HIT is to discontinue heparin and start a non-heparin anticoagulant, such as argatroban or fondaparinux, to prevent thrombosis while avoiding further platelet activation.

SBA 63: d) Hypertension

Hypertension is not a common side effect of anticoagulant therapy. The other options listed are potential side effects, with bleeding being the most significant concern.

SBA 64: c) Microangiopathic hemolytic anemia

Schistocytes, or fragmented red blood cells, are typically seen in microangiopathic hemolytic anemia, which includes conditions like TTP and DIC.

SBA 65: b) High platelet count

Essential thrombocythemia is a myeloproliferative disorder characterized by an abnormally high platelet count, which can lead to both bleeding and thrombotic complications.

SBA 66: c) Drug-induced thrombocytopenia

Drug-induced thrombocytopenia is the most common cause of thrombocytopenia in hospitalized patients, often resulting from the use of certain medications that affect platelet production or function.

SBA 67: c) Activated partial thromboplastin time (aPTT)

The aPTT test measures the intrinsic pathway of the coagulation cascade, which includes factors XII, XI, IX, and VIII.

SBA 68: c) Plasma exchange

Plasma exchange is the treatment of choice for severe TTP, as it removes the autoantibodies against ADAMTS13 and replenishes functional ADAMTS13 enzyme.

SBA 69: c) Vitamin K deficiency

Vitamin K deficiency leads to a decrease in the synthesis of vitamin K-dependent coagulation factors (II, VII, IX, and X), resulting in a prolonged PT.

SBA 70: d) Factor V Leiden mutation

The Factor V Leiden mutation is the most common cause of inherited thrombophilia, leading to resistance to activated protein C and an increased risk of venous thromboembolism.

SBA 71: e) Elevated white blood cell count

An elevated white blood cell count is not typically associated with APS. APS is characterized by recurrent miscarriages, venous and arterial thrombosis, and thrombocytopenia.

SBA 72: b) To mediate platelet adhesion to subendothelial collagen

The primary function of vWF is to mediate platelet adhesion to subendothelial collagen at the site of vascular injury, initiating the formation of a platelet plug.

SBA 73: b) Pulmonary embolism

A common complication of DVT is pulmonary embolism, where a blood clot dislodges and travels to the lungs, potentially causing life-threatening respiratory issues.

SBA 74: d) All of the above

The primary treatment for essential thrombocythemia may include hydroxyurea, aspirin, and anagrelide, which are used to reduce the risk of thrombosis and control symptoms.

SBA 75: d) Normal D-dimer levels

DIC is characterized by increased fibrin degradation products and elevated D-dimer levels due to widespread activation of the coagulation system and secondary fibrinolysis.

SBA 76: b) Chronic myeloid leukemia (CML)

The Philadelphia chromosome is a genetic abnormality found in the cancer cells of most patients with CML.

SBA 77: d) Diffuse large B-cell lymphoma

Diffuse large B-cell lymphoma is the most common subtype of non-Hodgkin lymphoma.

SBA78: c) Bence Jones proteins

Bence Jones proteins are light chains of immunoglobulins that are typically found in the urine of patients with multiple myeloma.

SBA 79: b) All-trans retinoic acid (ATRA)

ATRA, in combination with chemotherapy, is the primary treatment for APL and has significantly improved outcomes.

SBA 80: c) CD3

CD3 is a T-cell marker, whereas CD19, CD20, CD22, and CD79a are B-cell markers.

SBA 81: c) Painless lymphadenopathy

Painless enlargement of lymph nodes is the most common presenting symptom of Hodgkin lymphoma.

SBA 82: c) TP53

TP53 mutations are associated with poor prognosis in CLL and are found in a subset of patients.

SBA 83: c) Reed-Sternberg cell

The presence of Reed-Sternberg cells is diagnostic of Hodgkin lymphoma.

SBA 84: d) All of the above

Smoking, previous chemotherapy or radiation therapy, and certain genetic syndromes are risk factors for AML.

SBA 85: d) t(12;21)(p13;q22)

The translocation t(12;21)(p13;q22) is the most common cytogenetic abnormality in adult ALL.

SBA 86: a) Transformation to acute leukemia

MDS can progress to acute leukemia, particularly AML, in a subset of patients.

SBA 87: a) Signal transduction
CD20 plays a role in B-cell activation and differentiation through signal transduction.
SBA 88: d) Hypercalcemia
Hypercalcemia is not a typical symptom of CML. Common symptoms include fatigue, splenomegaly, easy bruising, and night sweats.
SBA 89: b) Bone pain
Bone pain, particularly in the back or ribs, is the most common presenting symptom of multiple myeloma due to bone lesions.
SBA 90: a) Hyperviscosity syndrome
Waldenström macroglobulinemia is characterized by the production of large amounts of IgM, leading to hyperviscosity syndrome.
SBA 91: c) Rituximab
Rituximab, a monoclonal antibody targeting CD20, is commonly used in the treatment of follicular lymphoma.
SBA 92: c) Acute lymphoblastic leukemia (ALL)
ALL is the most common type of leukemia in children and is highly treatable with a good prognosis.
SBA 93: c) Complex karyotype
A complex karyotype, defined as three or more chromosomal abnormalities, is associated with a poor prognosis in AML.
SBA 94: d) Hypertension
Hypertension is not a common side effect of chemotherapy. Common side effects include nausea, vomiting, hair loss, neuropathy, and myelosuppression.
SBA 95: c) Translocation t(8;14)(q24;q32)
Burkitt lymphoma is characterized by the translocation t(8;14)(q24;q32), which involves the c-myc gene on chromosome 8 and the immunoglobulin heavy chain locus on chromosome 14. This translocation leads to overexpression of the c-myc oncogene, which is a key factor in the development of Burkitt lymphoma.
SBA 96: d) Mutation in the JAK2 gene
Primary polycythemia, also known as polycythemia vera, is most commonly caused by a mutation in the JAK2 gene, which leads to uncontrolled red blood cell production.
SBA 97: d) Tachycardia
Tachycardia is not commonly associated with polycythemia vera. Common symptoms include headaches, dizziness, hypertension, and pruritus, especially after a hot shower or bath.
SBA 98: a) Thrombosis
The most common complication of secondary polycythemia is thrombosis due to increased blood viscosity and red blood cell mass.
SBA 99: d) Elevated red blood cell mass

Elevated red blood cell mass is a major diagnostic criterion for polycythemia vera, along with JAK2 mutation and low erythropoietin levels.

SBA 100: b) Phlebotomy

The initial treatment of choice for reducing hematocrit in polycythemia vera is phlebotomy, which involves removing blood from the body to decrease blood volume and red blood cell mass

SBA 101: e) Direct platelet production by myeloma cells

Multiple myeloma does not directly produce platelets. Thrombocytopenia in multiple myeloma is typically due to bone marrow infiltration by plasma cells, increased platelet destruction, nutritional deficiencies, or myelosuppressive chemotherapy.

SBA 102: c) Bone marrow replacement by malignant plasma cells

Anemia in multiple myeloma is primarily due to the replacement of normal bone marrow hematopoietic cells by malignant plasma cells, leading to decreased production of red blood cells.

SBA 103: c) Rouleaux formation

Rouleaux formation, which is the stacking of red blood cells resembling a stack of coins, is a characteristic finding on the peripheral blood smear of patients with multiple myeloma due to the high serum protein concentration.

SBA 104: e) Elevated serum creatinine

Elevated serum creatinine is a poor prognostic marker in multiple myeloma, indicating renal impairment which is often due to light chain deposition in the kidneys.

SBA 106: d) Thrombocytosis

Thrombocytosis, or an elevated platelet count, is not a common clinical feature of multiple myeloma. Patients with multiple myeloma more commonly experience bone pain, recurrent infections, weight loss, and anemia.

SBA 106: d) O+

O+ is the most common blood type globally, with about 37% of the population having this type. However, the distribution of blood types varies by region and ethnicity. For example, in some parts of Asia, B+ is more prevalent than O+.

SBA 107: e) O-

O- blood type can donate to any other blood type, because it does not have any antigens on the surface of the red blood cells that could trigger an immune response in the recipient. However, O- blood type is rare, with only about 7% of the population having this type.

SBA 108: c) AB+

AB+ blood type can receive from any other blood type, because it has both A and B antigens on the surface of the red blood cells, and therefore does not produce antibodies against either antigen. However, AB+ blood type is also rare, with only about 3% of the population having this type.

SBA 109: a) It is a protein on the surface of the red blood cells that determines the blood type.

The Rh factor, also known as the D antigen, is a protein that is present or absent on the surface of the red blood cells. People who have the Rh factor are Rh positive, and those who do not have it are Rh negative. The Rh factor is important for blood transfusion, because if a Rh-negative person receives Rh positive blood, their immune system will produce antibodies against the Rh factor and cause a hemolytic reaction.

SBA 110: c) Febrile reaction

A febrile reaction is a mild to moderate reaction that occurs when the recipient's immune system reacts to the donor's white blood cells or platelets. It is characterized by fever, chills, headache, and sometimes nausea and vomiting. It can be prevented by using leukocyte-reduced blood products, which have most of the white blood cells removed.

SBA 111: D) Transfusion-related acute lung injury (TRALI)

TRALI is a rare but life-threatening reaction that occurs when the recipient's immune system reacts to the donor's plasma proteins or antibodies. It is characterized by acute respiratory distress, hypoxemia, hypotension, and pulmonary edema. It can be prevented by using plasma-reduced blood products, which have most of the plasma removed.

SBA 112: c) Hepatitis C

Hepatitis C is a viral infection that affects the liver and can cause chronic inflammation, cirrhosis, and liver cancer. It is transmitted through contact with infected blood or body fluids. The risk of hepatitis C transmission through blood transfusion is very low, as all donated blood is screened for the virus. However, there is still a small chance of transmission due to the window period, which is the time between the infection and the detection of the virus in the blood.

SBA 113: a) HIV

HIV is a viral infection that affects the immune system and can cause acquired immunodeficiency syndrome (AIDS). It is transmitted through contact with infected blood or body fluids. The risk of HIV transmission through blood transfusion is extremely low, as all donated blood is screened for the virus and the window period is very short.

SBA 114: b) Packed red blood cells

Packed red blood cells are red blood cells that have been separated from plasma and other blood components. They are used to increase the oxygen-carrying capacity of the blood and to treat severe anemia. They have a shelf life of up to 42 days and can be stored at 2-6 degrees Celsius.

SBA 115: a) Whole blood

Whole blood is blood that has not been separated into its components. It is used to replace the blood volume and the oxygen-carrying capacity of the blood in patients with severe bleeding. It has a shelf life of up to 35 days and can be stored at 2-6 degrees Celsius.

SBA 116: c) Fresh frozen plasma

Fresh frozen plasma is plasma that has been separated from the blood cells and frozen within 8 hours of collection. It is used to provide clotting factors and to treat coagulation disorders. It has a shelf life of up to one year and can be stored at -18 degrees Celsius or below.

SBA 117: d) Platelets

Platelets are cell fragments that are involved in blood clotting and hemostasis. They are used to prevent or treat bleeding in patients with low platelet counts or platelet dysfunction. They have a shelf life of up to 5 days and can be stored at 20-24 degrees Celsius with gentle agitation.

SBA 118: e) Cryoprecipitate

Cryoprecipitate is a concentrated source of fibrinogen, factor VIII, factor XIII, von Willebrand factor, and fibronectin. It is used to treat bleeding in patients with hemophilia A, von Willebrand disease, or fibrinogen deficiency. It has a shelf life of up to one year and can be stored at -18 degrees Celsius or below.

SBA 119: b) Packed red blood cells

Sickle cell disease is a genetic disorder that causes the red blood cells to have an abnormal shape and function. It can cause chronic anemia, pain, infections, and organ damage. The treatment is to transfuse the patient with packed red blood cells that are matched for the patient's blood type and sickle cell phenotype.

SBA 120: a) Whole blood

Massive blood loss can cause hypovolemic shock, which is a life-threatening condition that occurs when the blood volume is too low to maintain adequate blood pressure and organ perfusion. The treatment is to transfuse the patient with whole blood, which can restore both the blood volume and the oxygen-carrying capacity of the blood.

SBA 121: c) Fresh frozen plasma

TTP is a rare disorder that causes the formation of microclots in the small blood vessels, resulting in hemolytic anemia, thrombocytopenia, fever, neurological symptoms, and kidney failure. It is caused by a deficiency or dysfunction of a plasma enzyme called ADAMTS13, which normally cleaves von Willebrand factor. The treatment is to transfuse the patient with fresh frozen plasma, which can provide the missing or defective enzyme and prevent further clotting.

SBA 122: c) Fresh frozen plasma

DIC is a condition that occurs when the coagulation system is activated inappropriately and excessively, leading to widespread clotting and bleeding. It is usually triggered by a severe infection, trauma, malignancy, or obstetric complication. The treatment is to transfuse the patient with fresh frozen plasma, which can provide the depleted clotting factors and inhibitors and restore the balance of the coagulation system.

SBA 123: d) Platelets

Acute leukemia is a cancer of the blood-forming cells in the bone marrow, which results in the production of abnormal and immature white blood cells. It can cause anemia, infection, and bleeding. The treatment is to transfuse the patient with platelets, which can prevent or treat bleeding due to low platelet counts or platelet dysfunction.

SBA 124: b) Packed red blood cells

Iron deficiency anemia is a common type of anemia that occurs when the body does not have enough iron to produce hemoglobin, the protein that carries oxygen in the red blood cells. It can cause fatigue, weakness, pallor, and shortness of breath. The treatment is to transfuse the patient with packed red blood cells, which can increase the hemoglobin level and improve the oxygen delivery to the tissues. However, blood transfusion is usually reserved for severe cases of iron deficiency anemia, and the underlying cause of the iron deficiency should also be addressed.

SBA 125: b) Packed red blood cells

This condition is called hemolytic disease of the newborn, and it can occur when the mother and the baby have incompatible blood types, such as Rh or ABO. The mother's antibodies cross the placenta and destroy the baby's red blood cells, causing anemia. The treatment is to transfuse the baby with packed red blood cells that match the baby's blood type and do not have the antigens that the mother's antibodies react to.

References

1. Cazzola, Mario. "Introduction to a Review Series on Normal and Pathologic Erythropoiesis." Blood 139.16 (2022): 2413-2414. doi: 10.1182/blood.2022015497

2. "Anaemia." World Health Organization (WHO), published November 2021. Accessed September 18, 2022. <https://www.who.int/health-topics/anaemia#tab=tab_1>

3. "Anemia - Diagnosis and treatment." Mayo Clinic, published May 11, 2023. Accessed September 18, 2022. <https://www.mayoclinic.org/diseases-conditions/anemia/diagnosis-treatment/drc-20351366>

4. Hoffbrand, AV, Moss, PAH, and Pettit, JE. Essential Haematology. 7th ed. Wiley Blackwell, 2015.

5. Kumar, Vinay, Abbas, Akik K., and Aster, Jon C. Robbins and Cotran Pathologic Basis of Disease. 9th ed. Elsevier, 2015.

6. McPherson, Richard A., and Pincus, Mark R. Henry's Clinical Diagnosis and Management by Laboratory Methods. 23rd ed. Elsevier, 2017.

7. Kunak, Rachel L., Rojiani, Ali, and Savage, Nancy M. "Educational Case: Acute Promyelocytic Leukemia With PML-RARA." Academic Pathology 6.3 (2019): e2374289519875647. doi: 10.1177/2374289519875647

8. 100 Questions & Answers About Leukemia. 4th ed. Jones & Bartlett Learning, 2017.

9. Leukemia: Principles and Practice of Therapy. Wiley-Blackwell, 2010.

10. Hoffman, Robert, et al. Hematology: Basic Principles and Practice. Elsevier Inc., 2017. 2374 p. doi: 10.1016/C2013-0-23355-9

11. Siegel, Theodore, Grisariu, Sorin, Avni, Benjamin, and Baehring, Jeffrey. "Neurolymphomatosis." In: Batchelor, Timothy, and DeAngelis, Linda, eds. Lymphoma and Leukemia of the Nervous System. New York, NY: Springer, 2012. pp. 219-229.

12. Leukemia: Methods and Protocols. Totowa, NJ: Humana Press; 2019.

13. Kurosawa S, Yamaguchi T, Miyawaki S, et al. Prognostic Factors and Outcomes of Adult Patients with Acute Myeloid Leukemia After First Relapse. Haematologica. 2010;95(11):1857-1864. doi:10.3324/haematol.2010.027516

14. Bellan C, Lazzi S, De Falco G, Nyongo A, Giordano A, Leoncini L. Burkitt's Lymphoma: New Insights Into Molecular Pathogenesis. J Clin Pathol. 2003;56(3):188-192. doi:10.1136/jcp.56.3.188

15. Schafer AI. Molecular Basis of the Diagnosis and Treatment of Polycythemia Vera and Essential Thrombocythemia. Blood. 2006;107(11):4214-4222. doi:10.1182/blood-2005-08-3526

16. Tefferi A, Barbui T. Polycythemia Vera: 2024 Update on Diagnosis, Risk-Stratification, and Management. Am J Hematol. 2023;98(9):1465-1487. doi:10.1002/ajh.27002

17. Raedler LA. Diagnosis and Management of Polycythemia Vera: Proceedings from a Multidisciplinary Roundtable. Am Health Drug Benefits. 2014;7(7 suppl 3):S36-S47.

18. Gerecke C, Fuhrmann S, Strifler S, Schmidt-Hieber M, Einsele H, Knop S. The Diagnosis and Treatment of Multiple Myeloma. Dtsch Arztebl Int. 2016;113(27-28):470-476. doi:10.3238/arztebl.2016.0470

19. Dean L. Blood Groups and Red Cell Antigens [Internet]. Bethesda (MD): National Center for Biotechnology Information (US); 2005. Available from: <https://www.ncbi.nlm.nih.gov/books/NBK2261/>

20. Yaddanapudi S, Yaddanapudi L. Indications for Blood and Blood Product Transfusion. Indian J Anaesth. 2014;58(5):538-542. doi:10.4103/0019-5049.144648

21. Papageorgiou C, Jourdi G, Adjambri E, et al. Disseminated Intravascular Coagulation: An Update on Pathogenesis, Diagnosis, and Therapeutic Strategies. Clin Appl Thromb Hemost. 2018;24(9_suppl):8S-28S. doi:10.1177/1076029618806424

22. Ddungu H, Krantz EM, Kajja I, et al. Transfusion Challenges in Patients with Hematological Malignancies in Sub-Saharan Africa: A Prospective Observational Study from the Uganda Cancer Institute. Sci Rep. 2020;10(1):2825. Published 2020 Feb 18. doi:10.1038/s41598-020-59773-y

23. Clark SF. Iron Deficiency Anemia: Diagnosis and Management. Curr Opin Gastroenterol. 2009;25(2):122-128. doi:10.1097/MOG.0b013e32831ef1cd

24. Hendrickson JE, Delaney M. Hemolytic Disease of the Fetus and Newborn: Modern Practice and Future Investigations. Transfus Med Rev. 2016;30(4):159-164. doi:10.1016/j.tmrv.2016.05.008

25. Miller KD, Goding Sauer A, Ortiz AP, et al. Cancer Statistics for Hispanics/Latinos, 2018. CA Cancer J Clin. 2018;68(6):425-445. doi:10.3322/caac.21494

SBQ 1: a) Iron deficiency anemia

Iron deficiency anemia is the most common type of anemia, and it occurs when the body does not have enough iron to produce hemoglobin. It is characterized by microcytic (low MCV), hypochromic (low MCH), and anisocytotic (high RDW) red blood cells. The serum iron level is low, the TIBC is high, and the ferritin level is low, reflecting the low iron stores in the body. The common causes of iron deficiency anemia include blood loss, dietary deficiency, malabsorption, and increased demand.

SBQ 2: c) Thalassemia

Thalassemia is a genetic disorder that affects the synthesis of the alpha or beta chains of hemoglobin. It is characterized by microcytic (low MCV), hypochromic (low MCH), and normocytic (normal RDW) red blood cells. The serum iron level, TIBC, and ferritin level are normal, reflecting the normal iron metabolism in the body. The peripheral blood smear shows target cells, which are red blood cells with a central dark area, and basophilic stippling, which are small blue dots in the cytoplasm of the red blood cells. The common causes of thalassemia include Mediterranean, African, or Asian ancestry.

SBQ 3: b) Anemia of chronic disease

Anemia of chronic disease is a type of anemia that occurs in the setting of chronic inflammation, infection, or malignancy. It is characterized by normocytic (normal MCV), normochromic (normal MCH), and normocytic (normal RDW) red blood cells. The serum iron level is low, the TIBC is low, and the ferritin level is high, reflecting the impaired iron utilization and release from the macrophages. The common causes of anemia of chronic disease include autoimmune disorders, chronic infections, and cancers.

SBQ 4: e) Vitamin B12 deficiency anemia

Vitamin B12 deficiency anemia is a type of anemia that occurs when the body does not have enough vitamin B12 to produce DNA and red blood cells. It is characterized by macrocytic (high MCV), normochromic (normal MCH), and anisocytotic (high RDW) red blood cells. The serum vitamin B12 level is low, and the serum folate level is normal, reflecting the specific deficiency of vitamin B12. The peripheral blood smear shows macrocytic and oval-shaped red blood cells and hypersegmented neutrophils, which are white blood cells with more than five lobes in the nucleus. The common causes of vitamin B12 deficiency anemia includes pernicious anemia, dietary deficiency, malabsorption, and drugs.

SBQ 5: d) Sideroblastic anemia

Sideroblastic anemia is a type of anemia that occurs when the body has a defect in the heme synthesis pathway, leading to the accumulation of iron in the mitochondria of the red blood cells. It is characterized by normocytic (normal MCV), normochromic (normal MCH), and normocytic (normal RDW) red blood cells. The serum iron level is high, the TIBC is low, and the ferritin level is high, reflecting the excess iron in the body. The bone marrow biopsy shows ringed sideroblasts, which are red blood cell precursors with iron-laden mitochondria surrounding the nucleus. The common causes of sideroblastic anemia include genetic mutations, drugs, toxins, and alcohol.

SBQ 6: e) Folate deficiency anemia

Folate deficiency anemia is a type of anemia that occurs when the body does not have enough folate to produce DNA and red blood cells. It is characterized by macrocytic (high MCV), normochromic (normal MCH), and anisocytotic (high RDW) red blood cells. The serum folate level is low and the serum vitamin B12 level is normal, reflecting the specific deficiency of folate. The peripheral blood smear shows macrocytic and oval-shaped red blood cells and hypersegmented neutrophils, which are white blood cells with more than five lobes in the nucleus. The common causes of folate deficiency anemia include dietary deficiency, malabsorption, drugs, and increased demand.

SBQ 7: e) Hemolytic anemia

Hemolytic anemia is a type of anemia that occurs when the red blood cells are destroyed faster than they are produced. It is characterized by normocytic (normal MCV), normochromic (normal MCH), and anisocytotic (high RDW) red blood cells. The serum iron level, TIBC, and ferritin level are normal, reflecting the normal iron metabolism in the body. The peripheral blood smear shows sickle-shaped red blood cells, which are red blood cells that have an abnormal shape and function due to a mutation in the beta chain of hemoglobin, and Howell-Jolly bodies, which are nuclear remnants in the red blood cells due to the absence of the spleen. The common causes of hemolytic anemia include inherited disorders, such as sickle cell disease, autoimmune disorders, infections, drugs, and toxins.

SBQ 8: e) Aplastic anemia

Aplastic anemia is a type of anemia that occurs when the bone marrow fails to produce enough blood cells. It is characterized by normocytic (normal MCV), normochromic (normal MCH), and normocytic (normal RDW) red blood cells. The serum iron level, TIBC, and ferritin level are normal, reflecting the normal iron metabolism in the body. The platelet count and the white blood cell count are also low, reflecting the pancytopenia (low blood cell counts) in the blood. The bone marrow biopsy shows hypocellularity and increased fat, reflecting the failure of the hematopoietic stem cells. The common causes of aplastic anemia include idiopathic, drugs, toxins, radiation, infections, and autoimmune disorders.

SBQ 9: e) Hemolytic anemia

Hemolytic anemia is a type of anemia that occurs when the red blood cells are destroyed faster than they are produced. It is characterized by normocytic (normal MCV), normochromic (normal MCH), and anisocytotic (high RDW) red blood cells. The serum iron level, TIBC, and ferritin level are normal, reflecting the normal iron metabolism in the body. The peripheral blood smear shows bite cells, which are red blood cells with a bite-like defect in the membrane, and Heinz bodies, which are precipitated hemoglobin in the red blood cells. The common causes of hemolytic anemia include inherited disorders, such as G6PD deficiency, autoimmune disorders, infections, drugs, and toxins.

SBQ 10: a) Iron deficiency anemia

Iron deficiency anemia is the most common type of anemia, and it occurs when the body does not have enough iron to produce hemoglobin. It is characterized by microcytic (low MCV), hypochromic (low MCH), and anisocytotic (high RDW) red blood cells. The serum iron level is low, the TIBC is high, and the ferritin level is low, reflecting the low iron stores in the body. The serum vitamin B12 level is normal and the serum folate level is low, reflecting the malabsorption of folate due to celiac disease. The common causes of iron deficiency anemia include blood loss, dietary deficiency, malabsorption, and increased demand.

SBQ 11: e) Vitamin B12 deficiency anemia

Vitamin B12 deficiency anemia is a type of anemia that occurs when the body does not have enough vitamin B12 to produce DNA and red blood cells. It is characterized by macrocytic (high MCV), normochromic (normal MCH), and anisocytotic (high RDW) red blood cells. The serum vitamin B12 level is low, and the serum folate level is normal, reflecting the specific deficiency of vitamin B12. The peripheral blood smear shows macrocytic and oval-shaped red blood cells and hypersegmented neutrophils, which are white blood cells with more than five lobes in the nucleus. The common causes of vitamin B12 deficiency anemia includes pernicious anemia, dietary deficiency, malabsorption, and drugs.

SBQ 12: e) Aplastic anemia

Aplastic anemia is a type of anemia that occurs when the bone marrow fails to produce enough blood cells. It is characterized by normocytic (normal MCV), normochromic (normal MCH), and normocytic (normal RDW) red blood cells. The serum iron level, TIBC, and ferritin level are normal, reflecting the normal iron metabolism in the body. The platelet count and the white blood cell count are also low, reflecting the pancytopenia (low blood cell counts) in the blood. The bone marrow biopsy shows increased blasts, which are immature blood cells that have not differentiated into mature blood cells. The common causes of aplastic anemia include idiopathic, drugs, toxins, radiation, infections, and autoimmune disorders.

SBQ 13: e) Hemolytic anemia

Hemolytic anemia is a type of anemia that occurs when the red blood cells are destroyed faster than they are produced. It is characterized by normocytic (normal MCV), normochromic (normal MCH), and anisocytotic (high RDW) red blood cells. The serum iron level, TIBC, and ferritin level are normal, reflecting the normal iron metabolism in the body. The peripheral blood smear shows spherocytes, which are red blood cells that have a spherical shape and lack the central pallor, and polychromasia, which is the presence of young and immature red blood cells that have a bluish tint. The common causes of hemolytic anemia include inherited disorders, such as hereditary spherocytosis, autoimmune disorders, infections, drugs, and toxins.

SBQ 14: a) Blood loss

Blood loss is the most common cause of iron deficiency anemia, especially in women of reproductive age. It can occur due to menstrual bleeding, gastrointestinal bleeding, trauma, surgery, or other sources of hemorrhage. Blood loss leads to a depletion of iron stores and a reduction of hemoglobin synthesis. The anemia is characterized by microcytic (low MCV), hypochromic (low MCH), and anisocytotic (high RDW) red blood cells. The serum iron level is low, the TIBC is high, and the ferritin level is low, reflecting the low iron stores in the body. The serum vitamin B12 level and the serum folate level are normal, reflecting the normal synthesis of DNA and red blood cells.

SBQ 15: e) Folate deficiency anemia

Folate deficiency anemia is a type of anemia that occurs when the body does not have enough folate to produce DNA and red blood cells. It is characterized by macrocytic (high MCV), normochromic (normal MCH), and anisocytotic (high RDW) red blood cells. The serum folate level is low and the serum vitamin B12 level is normal, reflecting the specific deficiency of folate. The peripheral blood smear shows macrocytic and oval-shaped red blood cells and hypersegmented neutrophils, which are white blood cells with more than five lobes in the nucleus. The common causes of folate deficiency anemia include dietary deficiency, malabsorption, drugs, and increased demand.

SBQ 16: e) Aplastic anemia

Aplastic anemia is a type of anemia that occurs when the bone marrow fails to produce enough blood cells. It is characterized by normocytic (normal MCV), normochromic (normal MCH), and normocytic (normal RDW) red blood cells. The serum iron level, TIBC, and ferritin level are normal, reflecting the normal iron metabolism in the body. The platelet count and the white blood cell count are also low, reflecting the pancytopenia (low blood cell counts) in the blood. The bone marrow biopsy shows hypocellularity and increased fat, reflecting the failure of the hematopoietic stem cells. The common causes of aplastic anemia include idiopathic, drugs, toxins, radiation, infections, and autoimmune disorders.

SBQ 17: e) Hemolytic anemia

Hemolytic anemia is a type of anemia that occurs when the red blood cells are destroyed faster than they are produced. It is characterized by normocytic (normal MCV), normochromic (normal MCH), and anisocytotic (high RDW) red blood cells. The serum iron level, TIBC, and ferritin level are normal, reflecting the normal iron metabolism in the body. The peripheral blood smear shows bite cells, which are red blood cells with a bite-like defect in the membrane, and Heinz bodies, which are precipitated hemoglobin in the red blood cells. The common causes of hemolytic anemia include inherited disorders, such as G6PD deficiency, autoimmune disorders, infections, drugs, and toxins.

SBQ 18: c) Infectious mononucleosis

Infectious mononucleosis is a viral infection caused by the Epstein-Barr virus (EBV) that affects the lymphoid tissues. It is characterized by fever, sore throat, lymphadenopathy, and splenomegaly. The complete blood count shows a leukocytosis (high white blood cell count) with a lymphocytosis (high lymphocyte count) and the presence of atypical lymphocytes, which are activated lymphocytes that have a large size and an indented nucleus. The diagnosis can be confirmed by a positive heterophile antibody test (Monospot test) or a positive EBV-specific antibody test.

SBQ 19: c) Disseminated tuberculosis.

Disseminated tuberculosis is a severe form of tuberculosis that occurs when the Mycobacterium tuberculosis bacteria spread from the lungs to other organs, such as the liver, spleen, bone marrow, and brain. It is more common in immunocompromised patients, such as those with HIV infection. It is characterized by fever, weight loss, night sweats, and organ dysfunction. The complete blood count shows a leukopenia (low white blood cell count) with a normal differential. The peripheral blood smear shows acid-fast bacilli, which are bacteria that retain the red color of the Ziehl-Neelsen stain after being washed with acid and alcohol. The diagnosis can be confirmed by a positive culture or polymerase chain reaction (PCR) test for M. tuberculosis.

SBQ 20: d) Hypereosinophilic syndrome

Hypereosinophilic syndrome is a rare disorder that occurs when the eosinophils, which are a type of white blood cell that are involved in allergic and inflammatory responses, are abnormally increased in the blood and tissues. It is characterized by recurrent infections, eczema, asthma, and organ damage. The complete blood count shows a leukocytosis (high white blood cell count) with an eosinophilia (high eosinophil count). The peripheral blood smear shows eosinophilia, which is the presence of more than 500 eosinophils/mm3 in the blood. The diagnosis can be confirmed by ruling out other causes of eosinophilia, such as infections, malignancies, or drugs.

SBQ 21: d) Richter transformation

Richter transformation is a rare complication of chronic lymphocytic leukemia that occurs when the disease transforms into a more aggressive form of lymphoma, usually diffuse large B-cell lymphoma. It is characterized by a rapid increase in the white blood cell count, the appearance of large, immature lymphocytes in the blood and bone marrow, and the development of lymph node enlargement, organomegaly, and constitutional symptoms. The diagnosis can be confirmed by a lymph node biopsy.

SBQ 22: d) Hypereosinophilic syndrome
Hypereosinophilic syndrome is a rare disorder that occurs when the
eosinophils, which are a type of white blood cell that are involved in allergic
and inflammatory responses, are abnormally increased in the blood and
tissues. It is characterized by recurrent infections, eczema, asthma, and
organ damage. The complete blood count shows a leukocytosis (high white
blood cell count) with an eosinophilia (high eosinophil count). The
peripheral blood smear shows eosinophilia, which is the presence of more
than 500 eosinophils/mm3 in the blood. The diagnosis can be confirmed by
ruling out other causes of eosinophilia, such as infections, malignancies, or
drugs.
SBQ 23: b) Chronic myeloid leukemia
Chronic myeloid leukemia is a type of leukemia that occurs when the bone
marrow produces too many myeloid cells, which are the precursors of
neutrophils, eosinophils, basophils, and monocytes. It is caused by a genetic
mutation that results in the formation of the Philadelphia chromosome,
which is a translocation between chromosomes 9 and 22. It is characterized
by a leukocytosis (high white blood cell count) with a neutrophilia (high
neutrophil count) and the presence of immature myeloid cells in the blood
and bone marrow. The serum uric acid level is high, and the serum creatinine
level is high, reflecting the increased cell turnover and the impaired renal
function. The diagnosis can be confirmed by a cytogenetic analysis or a
molecular test for the BCR-ABL gene.
SBQ 24: c) Myelodysplastic syndrome
Myelodysplastic syndrome is a group of disorders that occur when the bone
marrow produces abnormal and dysfunctional blood cells. It is characterized
by a pancytopenia (low blood cell counts) with a normal or hypercellular
bone marrow. The peripheral blood smear shows pancytopenia, which is the
presence of low red blood cell, white blood cell, and platelet counts in the
blood. The diagnosis can be confirmed by a bone marrow biopsy and a
cytogenetic analysis.
SBQ 25: b) Acute myeloid leukemia

Acute myeloid leukemia is a type of leukemia that occurs when the bone
marrow produces too many myeloid cells, which are the precursors of
neutrophils, eosinophils, basophils, and monocytes. It is characterized by a
leukocytosis (high white blood cell count) with a predominance of blasts,
which are immature myeloid cells that have not differentiated into mature
myeloid cells. The peripheral blood smear shows large, immature cells with
high nuclear-to-cytoplasmic ratio and prominent nucleoli. The diagnosis can
be confirmed by a bone marrow biopsy and a flow cytometry or
immunophenotyping test. The common risk factors for acute myeloid
leukemia include genetic syndromes, such as Down syndrome, exposure to
radiation or chemicals, and previous chemotherapy or radiation therapy.

SBQ 26: c) Chronic lymphocytic leukemia

Chronic lymphocytic leukemia is a type of leukemia that occurs when the bone marrow produces too many lymphocytes, which are a type of white blood cell that are involved in the immune system. It is characterized by a leukocytosis (high white blood cell count) with a predominance of small, mature lymphocytes that have a narrow rim of cytoplasm and a dense nucleus. The peripheral blood smear shows small, mature lymphocytes with a narrow rim of cytoplasm and a dense nucleus. The diagnosis can be confirmed by a flow cytometry or immunophenotyping test. The common risk factors for chronic lymphocytic leukemia include age, sex, family history, and autoimmune disorders.

SBQ 27: e) Hairy cell leukemia

Hairy cell leukemia is a rare type of leukemia that occurs when the bone marrow produces too many B lymphocytes, which are a type of white blood cell that produce antibodies. It is characterized by a leukocytosis (high white blood cell count) with a predominance of hairy cells, which are lymphocytes with cytoplasmic projections that give them a hairy appearance. The peripheral blood smear shows hairy cells, which are lymphocytes with cytoplasmic projections. The diagnosis can be confirmed by a bone marrow biopsy and a flow cytometry or immunophenotyping test. The common risk factors for hairy cell leukemia include age, sex, and viral infections, such as hepatitis C.

SBQ 28: b) Acute myeloid leukemia

Acute myeloid leukemia is a type of leukemia that occurs when the bone marrow produces too many myeloid cells, which are the precursors of neutrophils, eosinophils, basophils, and monocytes. It is characterized by a leukocytosis (high white blood cell count) with a predominance of blasts, which are immature myeloid cells that have not differentiated into mature myeloid cells. The peripheral blood smear shows large, immature cells with high nuclear-to-cytoplasmic ratio and prominent nucleoli. The diagnosis can be confirmed by a bone marrow biopsy and a flow cytometry or immunophenotyping test. The common risk factors for acute myeloid leukemia include genetic syndromes, such as Down syndrome, exposure to radiation or chemicals, and previous chemotherapy or radiation therapy.

SBQ 29: c) Chronic lymphocytic leukemia

Chronic lymphocytic leukemia is a type of leukemia that occurs when the bone marrow produces too many lymphocytes, which are a type of white blood cell that are involved in the immune system. It is characterized by a leukocytosis (high white blood cell count) with a predominance of small, mature lymphocytes that have a narrow rim of cytoplasm and a dense nucleus. The peripheral blood smear shows small, mature lymphocytes with a narrow rim of cytoplasm and a dense nucleus. The diagnosis can be confirmed by a flow cytometry or immunophenotyping test. The common risk factors for chronic lymphocytic leukemia include age, sex, family history, and autoimmune disorders.

SBQ 30: e) Hairy cell leukemia

Hairy cell leukemia is a rare type of leukemia that occurs when the bone marrow produces too many B lymphocytes, which are a type of white blood cell that produce antibodies. It is characterized by a leukocytosis (high white blood cell count) with a predominance of hairy cells, which are lymphocytes with cytoplasmic projections that give them a hairy appearance. The peripheral blood smear shows hairy cells, which are lymphocytes with cytoplasmic projections. The diagnosis can be confirmed by a bone marrow biopsy and a flow cytometry or immunophenotyping test. The common risk factors for hairy cell leukemia include age, sex, and viral infections, such as hepatitis C.

SBQ 31: C) Myelodysplastic syndrome

Myelodysplastic syndrome is a group of disorders that occur when the bone marrow produces abnormal and dysfunctional blood cells. It is characterized by a pancytopenia (low blood cell counts) with a normal or hypercellular bone marrow. The peripheral blood smear shows pancytopenia, which is the presence of low red blood cell, white blood cell, and platelet counts in the blood. The diagnosis can be confirmed by a bone marrow biopsy and a cytogenetic analysis. The common risk factors for myelodysplastic syndrome include age, exposure to radiation or chemicals, and previous chemotherapy or radiation therapy.

SBQ 32: D) Chronic myeloid leukemia

Chronic myeloid leukemia is a type of leukemia that occurs when the bone marrow produces too many myeloid cells, which are the precursors of neutrophils, eosinophils, basophils, and monocytes. It is caused by a genetic mutation that results in the formation of the Philadelphia chromosome, which is a translocation between chromosomes 9 and 22. It is characterized by a leukocytosis (high white blood cell count) with a basophilia (high basophil count) and the presence of immature myeloid cells in the blood and bone marrow. The peripheral blood smear shows basophilia and immature myeloid cells. The diagnosis can be confirmed by a cytogenetic analysis or a molecular test for the BCR-ABL gene. The common risk factors for chronic myeloid leukemia include age, sex, and exposure to radiation or chemicals.

SBQ 33: a) Hodgkin lymphoma

Hodgkin lymphoma is a type of lymphoma that is characterized by the presence of Reed-Sternberg cells, which are derived from abnormal B lymphocytes. It typically affects young adults and presents with painless enlargement of lymph nodes, especially in the neck, chest, and abdomen. It can also cause systemic symptoms, such as fever, night sweats, weight loss, and itching. The diagnosis can be confirmed by a lymph node biopsy that shows Reed-Sternberg cells and a characteristic histological pattern.

SBQ 34: b) Non-Hodgkin lymphoma

Non-Hodgkin lymphoma is a heterogeneous group of lymphomas that arise from abnormal B or T lymphocytes. The patient's clinical and laboratory features are consistent with Waldenstrom macroglobulinemia, which is a type of non-Hodgkin lymphoma that involves the production of IgM by lymphoplasmacytic cells. It typically affects older adults and presents with fatigue, anemia, splenomegaly, and hyperviscosity syndrome. The diagnosis can be confirmed by a bone marrow biopsy that shows infiltration of lymphoplasmacytic cells and a serum protein electrophoresis that shows a monoclonal spike of IgM.

SBQ 35: b) Non-Hodgkin lymphoma

Non-Hodgkin lymphoma is a heterogeneous group of lymphomas that arise from abnormal B or T lymphocytes. The patient's clinical and laboratory features are consistent with follicular lymphoma, which is a type of non-Hodgkin lymphoma that involves the proliferation of small, cleaved B cells that form follicular structures in the lymph nodes. It typically affects middle-aged adults and presents with painless lymphadenopathy, often in the abdomen. It can also cause systemic symptoms, such as fever, weight loss, and night sweats. The diagnosis can be confirmed by a lymph node biopsy that shows small, cleaved cells with irregular nuclei and scant cytoplasm and a characteristic immunophenotype of CD20, CD10, and BCL-6.

SBQ 36: a) Hodgkin lymphoma

Hodgkin lymphoma is a type of lymphoma that is characterized by the presence of Reed-Sternberg cells, which are derived from abnormal B lymphocytes. It typically affects young adults and presents with painless enlargement of lymph nodes, especially in the neck, chest, and abdomen. It can also cause systemic symptoms, such as fever, night sweats, weight loss, and itching. The diagnosis can be confirmed by a lymph node biopsy that shows Reed-Sternberg cells and a characteristic histological pattern. The patient's clinical and laboratory features are consistent with nodular sclerosis Hodgkin lymphoma, which is a subtype of Hodgkin lymphoma that involves the formation of fibrous bands in the lymph nodes and the presence of large, atypical cells with multilobed nuclei and prominent nucleoli. It typically affects young women and presents with mediastinal or cervical lymphadenopathy. It has a characteristic immunophenotype of CD30, CD15, and PAX5.

SBQ 37: d) Chronic lymphocytic leukemia

Chronic lymphocytic leukemia (CLL) is a type of leukemia that occurs when the bone marrow produces too many small, mature B lymphocytes. It is characterized by lymphocytosis, which is a high lymphocyte count in the peripheral blood, and lymphadenopathy, which is enlargement of lymph nodes. It typically affects older adults and presents with fatigue, anemia, and recurrent infections. It can also cause autoimmune complications, such as hemolytic anemia and thrombocytopenia. The diagnosis can be confirmed by a peripheral blood smear that shows small, mature lymphocytes with round nuclei and clumped chromatin and a lymph node biopsy that shows diffuse infiltration of small, mature lymphocytes with round nuclei and clumped chromatin. It has a characteristic immunophenotype of CD20, CD5, and CD23.

SBQ 38: a) Primary polycythemia

Primary polycythemia, also known as polycythemia vera, is a type of myeloproliferative disorder that occurs when the bone marrow produces too many red blood cells. It is characterized by a high hemoglobin, hematocrit, and red blood cell count, with a low serum erythropoietin level. The common risk factors for primary polycythemia include age, sex, and genetic mutations. The common symptoms include headache, dizziness, blurred vision, itching, and thrombosis.

SBQ 39: b) Secondary polycythemia due to hypoxia

Secondary polycythemia due to hypoxia is a type of polycythemia that occurs when the body produces more red blood cells in response to low oxygen levels. It is characterized by a high hemoglobin, hematocrit, and red blood cell count, with a high serum erythropoietin level. The common causes of hypoxia include lung diseases, such as COPD, heart diseases, such as congenital heart defects, and high altitude. The common symptoms include fatigue, dyspnea, cyanosis, and clubbing.

SBQ 40: c) Secondary polycythemia due to erythropoietin-producing tumor

Secondary polycythemia due to erythropoietin-producing tumor is a type of polycythemia that occurs when a tumor produces excess erythropoietin, which stimulates the bone marrow to produce more red blood cells. It is characterized by a high hemoglobin, hematocrit, and red blood cell count, with a high serum erythropoietin level. The common tumors that produce erythropoietin include renal cell carcinoma, hepatocellular carcinoma, and pheochromocytoma. The common symptoms include abdominal pain, weight loss, night sweats, and paraneoplastic syndromes.

SBQ 41: d) Secondary polycythemia due to dehydration

Secondary polycythemia due to dehydration is a type of polycythemia that occurs when the body loses fluid, which causes the blood to become more concentrated. It is characterized by a high hemoglobin, hematocrit, and red blood cell count, with a normal serum erythropoietin level. The common causes of dehydration include diabetes mellitus, diuretic therapy, vomiting, diarrhea, and excessive sweating. The common symptoms include weakness, confusion, constipation, and dry skin.

SBQ 42: e) Secondary polycythemia due to testosterone therapy

Secondary polycythemia due to testosterone therapy is a type of polycythemia that occurs when exogenous testosterone stimulates the bone marrow to produce more red blood cells. It is characterized by a high hemoglobin, hematocrit, and red blood cell count, with a normal serum erythropoietin level. The common indications for testosterone therapy include hypogonadism, male menopause, and gender dysphoria. The common side effects include erectile dysfunction, mood swings, decreased muscle mass, and increased risk of cardiovascular events.

SBQ 43: a) Multiple myeloma

Multiple myeloma is a type of plasma cell neoplasm that occurs when the bone marrow produces too many abnormal plasma cells, which are a type of white blood cell that produce antibodies. It is characterized by a monoclonal spike of immunoglobulin (Ig) in the serum or urine, bone lesions, anemia, renal insufficiency, hypercalcemia, and increased risk of infections. The diagnosis can be confirmed by a bone marrow biopsy that shows more than 10% plasma cells or a plasmacytoma (a single mass of plasma cells).

SBQ 44: b) Amyloidosis

Amyloidosis is a condition that occurs when abnormal proteins, such as immunoglobulin light chains, accumulate in various organs and tissues, causing damage and dysfunction. It is a common complication of multiple myeloma, especially when the monoclonal spike is of IgA or Ig D type. It is characterized by fatigue, bruising, recurrent infections, nephrotic syndrome, cardiomyopathy, peripheral neuropathy, and hepatosplenomegaly. The diagnosis can be confirmed by a tissue biopsy that shows apple-green birefringence under polarized light after staining with Congo red.

SBQ 45: a) Bone resorption due to osteoclast activation by cytokines from plasma cells

Hypercalcemia is a condition that occurs when the serum calcium level is above the normal range of 8.5 to 10.5 mg/dL. It is a common complication of multiple myeloma, affecting up to 30% of patients. It is caused by bone resorption due to osteoclast activation by cytokines, such as interleukin-1 (IL-1), interleukin-6 (IL-6), and tumor necrosis factor-alpha (TNF-alpha), from plasma cells. It is characterized by back pain, constipation, confusion, polyuria, polydipsia, and cardiac arrhythmias. The diagnosis can be confirmed by a serum calcium level above 11 mg/dL and a low serum phosphate level.

SBQ 46: a) Hyperviscosity syndrome

Hyperviscosity syndrome is a condition that occurs when the blood becomes too thick and viscous due to the presence of high levels of immunoglobulins, especially IgM, which is a large and pentameric molecule. It is a rare complication of multiple myeloma, affecting less than 5% of patients. It is characterized by blurred vision, headache, bleeding gums, dizziness, dyspnea, and stroke. The diagnosis can be confirmed by a serum viscosity above 4 centipoise and a fundoscopic examination that shows dilated and tortuous retinal veins, retinal hemorrhages, and papilledema.

SBQ 47: d) Tumor lysis syndrome

Tumor lysis syndrome is a condition that occurs when the rapid breakdown of tumor cells, such as plasma cells, releases large amounts of intracellular contents, such as uric acid, potassium, phosphate, and calcium, into the bloodstream. It is a rare but serious complication of multiple myeloma, especially after chemotherapy. It is characterized by hyperuricemia, hyperkalemia, hyperphosphatemia, hypocalcemia, and acute kidney injury. The diagnosis can be confirmed by a serum uric acid level above 8 mg/dL, a serum potassium level above 6 mEq/L, a serum phosphate level above 4.5 mg/dL, a serum calcium level below 7 mg/dL, and a serum creatinine level above 1.5 times the baseline.

SBQ 48: a) Glanzmann thrombasthenia

Glanzmann thrombasthenia is a rare inherited disorder of platelet function that is caused by a defect or deficiency of glycoprotein IIb/IIIa, which is a receptor for fibrinogen and other adhesive molecules on the platelet surface. It is characterized by mucocutaneous bleeding, such as bruising, epistaxis, and menorrhagia, and normal platelet count and morphology. The bleeding time is prolonged, but the coagulation tests are normal. The platelet aggregation test shows normal response to ristocetin, which activates von Willebrand factor, but impaired response to ADP, collagen, and epinephrine, which activate glycoprotein IIb/IIIa.

SBQ 49: e) Carcinoid syndrome

Carcinoid syndrome is a condition that occurs when a neuroendocrine tumor, usually located in the gastrointestinal tract or the lung, secretes excessive amounts of serotonin and other vasoactive substances into the bloodstream. It is characterized by flushing, diarrhea, bronchospasm, and right-sided valvular heart disease. It can also cause thrombosis, especially in the mesenteric and pulmonary circulation, due to the activation of platelets by serotonin. The platelet count and morphology are normal, but the platelet function may be impaired. The plasma serotonin level is elevated, and the urine 5-hydroxyindoleacetic acid (5-HIAA) level is also increased.

SBQ 50: a) Immune thrombocytopenic purpura

Immune thrombocytopenic purpura (ITP) is a type of autoimmune disorder that occurs when antibodies bind to platelets and cause their destruction by the spleen or the liver. It is characterized by isolated thrombocytopenia, which is a low platelet count without any other blood cell abnormalities. It can be triggered by infections, drugs, or other autoimmune diseases, such as systemic lupus erythematosus. The bleeding manifestations include petechiae, purpura, and mucosal bleeding. The coagulation tests are normal, and the peripheral blood smear shows no platelet clumps or schistocytes, which are fragmented red blood cells. The direct and indirect antiglobulin tests are negative, ruling out immune hemolysis. The platelet-associated IgG level is elevated, indicating the presence of anti-platelet antibodies.

SBQ 51: a) Glanzmann thrombasthenia

Glanzmann thrombasthenia is a rare inherited disorder of platelet function that is caused by a defect or deficiency of glycoprotein IIb/IIIa, which is a receptor for fibrinogen and other adhesive molecules on the platelet surface. It is characterized by mucocutaneous bleeding, such as epistaxis, gingival bleeding, and hematuria, and normal platelet count and morphology. The bleeding time is prolonged, but the coagulation tests are normal. The platelet aggregation test shows normal response to ristocetin, which activates von Willebrand factor, but absent response to ADP, collagen, epinephrine, and arachidonic acid, which activate glycoprotein IIb/IIIa.

SBQ 52: e) Drug-induced thrombocytopenia

Drug-induced thrombocytopenia is a type of acquired thrombocytopenia that occurs when certain drugs, such as heparin, quinine, or sulfonamides, bind to platelets and cause their destruction by the immune system. It is characterized by isolated thrombocytopenia, which is a low platelet count without any other blood cell abnormalities. It can occur within hours or days of drug exposure, and usually resolves after drug withdrawal. The bleeding manifestations include petechiae, purpura, and ecchymoses. The coagulation tests are normal, and the peripheral blood smear shows no platelet clumps or schistocytes, which are fragmented red blood cells. The direct and indirect antiglobulin tests are negative, ruling out immune hemolysis. The platelet-associated IgG level is normal, indicating the absence of anti-platelet antibodies.

SBQ 53: e) Uremic platelet dysfunction

Uremic platelet dysfunction is a type of acquired platelet dysfunction that occurs when the accumulation of urea and other metabolic waste products in the blood, due to renal failure, interferes with platelet function. It is characterized by mucocutaneous bleeding, such as epistaxis, gingival bleeding, and gastrointestinal bleeding, and normal or mildly reduced platelet count. The bleeding time is prolonged, but the coagulation tests are normal. The platelet aggregation test shows impaired response to all agonists, such as ADP, collagen, epinephrine, and ristocetin. The serum creatinine level is elevated, reflecting the impaired renal function.

SBQ 54: a) Essential thrombocythemia

Essential thrombocythemia is a type of myeloproliferative disorder that occurs when the bone marrow produces too many platelets. It is characterized by thrombocytosis, which is a high platelet count above 450,000/mm3, and increased risk of thrombosis and bleeding. The thrombosis can affect the arterial or venous circulation, and cause complications such as deep vein thrombosis, pulmonary embolism, stroke, and myocardial infarction. The bleeding can occur due to platelet dysfunction or acquired von Willebrand disease. The coagulation tests are normal, and the platelet aggregation test shows normal response to all agonists. The bone marrow biopsy shows increased number and size of megakaryocytes, which are the precursors of platelets.

SBQ 55: d) Aspirin-induced platelet dysfunction

Aspirin-induced platelet dysfunction is a type of acquired platelet dysfunction that occurs when aspirin, or other nonsteroidal anti-inflammatory drugs (NSAIDs), inhibit the cyclooxygenase (COX) enzyme in platelets, which is responsible for the synthesis of thromboxane A2, a potent platelet activator and vasoconstrictor. It is characterized by mucocutaneous bleeding, such as bruising, epistaxis, and hematuria, and normal platelet count and morphology. The bleeding time is prolonged, but the coagulation tests are normal. The platelet aggregation test shows normal response to ristocetin, which activates von Willebrand factor, but reduced response to ADP, collagen, epinephrine, and arachidonic acid, which activate thromboxane A2.

SBQ 56: c) von Willebrand disease

von Willebrand disease is the most common inherited bleeding disorder, affecting about 1% of the population. It is caused by a deficiency or dysfunction of von Willebrand factor, which is a protein that binds to platelets and factor VIII and mediates their adhesion to the injured blood vessel wall. It is characterized by mucocutaneous bleeding, such as menorrhagia, epistaxis, and bruising, and normal platelet count and morphology. The bleeding time is prolonged, but the coagulation tests are normal. The diagnosis can be confirmed by measuring the von Willebrand factor antigen and activity levels, which are low in most cases.

SBQ 57: a) Factor V Leiden

Factor V Leiden is the most common inherited thrombophilia, affecting about 5% of the Caucasian population. It is caused by a mutation in the factor V gene that renders it resistant to the inactivation by activated protein C, which is a natural anticoagulant that inhibits factors Va and VIIIa. It is characterized by a hypercoagulable state, which increases the risk of venous thromboembolism, such as deep vein thrombosis and pulmonary embolism. The coagulation tests are normal, but the plasma D-dimer level is elevated, indicating the presence of fibrin degradation products. The diagnosis can be confirmed by genetic testing or by measuring the activated protein C resistance ratio, which is low in most cases.

SBQ 58: a) Immune thrombocytopenic purpura

Immune thrombocytopenic purpura (ITP) is a type of autoimmune disorder that occurs when antibodies bind to platelets and cause their destruction by the spleen or the liver. It is characterized by isolated thrombocytopenia, which is a low platelet count without any other blood cell abnormalities. It can be triggered by infections, drugs, or other autoimmune diseases, such as systemic lupus erythematosus. The bleeding manifestations include petechiae, purpura, and mucosal bleeding. The coagulation tests are normal, and the peripheral blood smear shows no platelet clumps or schistocytes, which are fragmented red blood cells. The direct and indirect antiglobulin tests are negative, ruling out immune hemolysis. The platelet-associated IgG level is elevated, indicating the presence of anti-platelet antibodies.

SBQ 59: e) Uremic platelet dysfunction

Uremic platelet dysfunction is a type of acquired platelet dysfunction that occurs when the accumulation of urea and other metabolic waste products in the blood, due to renal failure, interferes with platelet function. It is characterized by mucocutaneous bleeding, such as epistaxis, gingival bleeding, and gastrointestinal bleeding, and normal or mildly reduced platelet count. The bleeding time is prolonged, but the coagulation tests are normal. The platelet aggregation test shows impaired response to all agonists, such as ADP, collagen, epinephrine, and ristocetin. The serum creatinine level is elevated, reflecting the impaired renal function.

SBQ 60: e) Antiphospholipid syndrome

Antiphospholipid syndrome is a type of acquired thrombophilia that occurs when antibodies bind to phospholipids or phospholipid-binding proteins, such as beta-2 glycoprotein I, and interfere with the normal function of the coagulation system. It is characterized by a hypercoagulable state, which increases the risk of arterial and venous thrombosis, as well as pregnancy complications, such as miscarriage, pre-eclampsia, and intrauterine growth restriction. The coagulation tests are normal, but the plasma D-dimer level is elevated, indicating the presence of fibrin degradation products. The diagnosis can be confirmed by the presence of anticardiolipin antibodies or lupus anticoagulant, which are two types of antiphospholipid antibodies, in the blood.

SBQ 61: a) Hemophilia A

Hemophilia A is the most common inherited bleeding disorder, affecting about 1 in 5,000 male births. It is caused by a deficiency or dysfunction of factor VIII, which is a coagulation factor that participates in the intrinsic pathway of the coagulation cascade. It is characterized by deep tissue bleeding, such as hemarthrosis, muscle hematoma, and retroperitoneal bleeding, and prolonged bleeding after minor trauma or surgery. The bleeding time is normal, but the prothrombin time is normal, and the activated partial thromboplastin time is prolonged, reflecting the defect in the intrinsic pathway. The diagnosis can be confirmed by measuring the factor VIII activity level, which is low in most cases.

SBQ 62: e) Antiphospholipid syndrome

Antiphospholipid syndrome is a type of acquired thrombophilia that occurs when antibodies bind to phospholipids or phospholipid-binding proteins, such as beta-2 glycoprotein I, and interfere with the normal function of the coagulation system. It is characterized by a hypercoagulable state, which increases the risk of arterial and venous thrombosis, as well as pregnancy complications, such as miscarriage, fetal growth restriction, placental abruption, and pre-eclampsia. The coagulation tests are normal, but the plasma D-dimer level may be elevated, indicating the presence of fibrin degradation products. The diagnosis can be confirmed by the presence of anticardiolipin antibodies or lupus anticoagulant, which are two types of antiphospholipid antibodies, in the blood.

SBQ 63: c) Disseminated intravascular coagulation

Disseminated intravascular coagulation (DIC) is a type of acquired coagulation disorder that occurs when the coagulation system is abnormally activated throughout the circulation, leading to the formation of microthrombi and the consumption of coagulation factors and platelets. It is usually triggered by a severe systemic condition, such as sepsis, trauma, malignancy, or obstetric complications. It is characterized by bleeding from multiple sites, such as skin, mucous membranes, and catheter sites, and organ dysfunction, such as renal failure, respiratory distress, and shock. The coagulation tests are prolonged, and the plasma D-dimer level is elevated, indicating the presence of fibrin degradation products. The peripheral blood smear shows platelet clumps and schistocytes, which are fragmented red blood cells. The fibrinogen level is low, reflecting the consumption of coagulation factors.

SBQ 64: d) Aspirin-induced platelet dysfunction

Aspirin-induced platelet dysfunction is a type of acquired platelet dysfunction that occurs when aspirin, or other nonsteroidal anti-inflammatory drugs (NSAIDs), inhibit the cyclooxygenase (COX) enzyme in platelets, which is responsible for the synthesis of thromboxane A2, a potent platelet activator and vasoconstrictor. It is characterized by mucocutaneous bleeding, such as epistaxis, gingival bleeding, and gastrointestinal bleeding, and normal platelet count and morphology. The bleeding time is prolonged, but the coagulation tests are normal. The plasma D-dimer level is normal, indicating the absence of fibrin degradation products. The fibrinogen level is normal, reflecting the normal synthesis of coagulation factors.

SBQ 65: d) Antithrombin deficiency

Antithrombin deficiency is a rare inherited or acquired thrombophilia that occurs when antithrombin, which is a natural anticoagulant that inhibits thrombin and other coagulation factors, is deficient or dysfunctional. It is characterized by a hypercoagulable state, which increases the risk of venous thromboembolism, such as deep vein thrombosis and pulmonary embolism. The coagulation tests are normal, but the plasma D-dimer level is elevated, indicating the presence of fibrin degradation products. The diagnosis can be confirmed by measuring the antithrombin activity level, which is low in most cases.

SBQ 66: d) Record the patient's vital signs and urine output.

The nurse should record the patient's baseline vital signs and urine output before starting the transfusion, as well as during and after the transfusion, to monitor for any signs of transfusion reactions, such as fever, chills, rash, dyspnea, hypotension, or hemoglobinuria. The nurse should obtain informed consent from the patient or a legal representative before obtaining the blood unit from the blood bank, not before starting the transfusion. The nurse should not administer any medications to the patient without a prescription from the health care provider, and only if the patient has a history of allergic or febrile reactions to blood transfusions. The nurse should flush the intravenous line with normal saline before and after the transfusion, not before starting the transfusion.

SBQ 67: e) Through a separate intravenous line from the blood transfusion. The nurse should administer the medication through a separate intravenous line from the blood transfusion, to avoid any incompatibility or interference with the blood product. The nurse should not administer the medication through the same intravenous line as the blood transfusion, as this could worsen the reaction or cause hemolysis. The nurse should not dilute the medication with normal saline, as this could reduce its effectiveness or cause fluid overload. The nurse should flush the intravenous line with normal saline before and after administering the medication, to ensure its delivery and prevent any precipitation or irritation.

SBQ 68: b) Febrile nonhemolytic reaction

The patient's reaction is most likely a febrile nonhemolytic reaction, which is caused by the recipient's antibodies reacting to the donor's leukocytes or cytokines. It is characterized by fever, chills, and rigors, and usually occurs within 2 hours of the transfusion. It is the most common type of transfusion reaction, especially with platelet transfusions. The patient's reaction is unlikely to be an acute hemolytic reaction, which is caused by the recipient's antibodies reacting to the donor's red blood cells. It is characterized by fever, chills, flank pain, hemoglobinuria, and shock, and usually occurs within minutes of the transfusion. It is the most serious and potentially fatal type of transfusion reaction. The patient's reaction is unlikely to be an allergic reaction, which is caused by the recipient's antibodies reacting to the donor's plasma proteins. It is characterized by urticaria, pruritus, flushing, and angioedema, and usually occurs within minutes of the transfusion. It is the most common type of transfusion reaction, especially with plasma transfusions. The patient's reaction is unlikely to be due to bacterial contamination, which is caused by the presence of bacteria in the blood product. It is characterized by fever, chills, hypotension, and septic shock, and usually occurs within minutes of the transfusion. It is the most common cause of transfusion-related mortality.

SBQ 69: b) 4 hours

The nurse should ensure that the transfusion is completed within 4 hours of obtaining the blood unit from the blood bank, to minimize the risk of bacterial growth and deterioration of the blood components. The nurse should not exceed this time limit, as this could compromise the safety and efficacy of the blood product. The nurse should not complete the transfusion too quickly, as this could cause fluid overload or circulatory overload. The nurse should administer the blood product at a rate of 2 to 4 mL/kg/hour, depending on the patient's condition and tolerance.

SBQ 70: a) Factor VIII

Cryoprecipitate is a blood product that contains high concentrations of factor VIII, as well as fibrinogen, von Willebrand factor, and factor XIII. It is used to treat hemophilia A, which is a bleeding disorder caused by a deficiency or dysfunction of factor VIII. It is also used to treat von Willebrand disease, which is a bleeding disorder caused by a deficiency or dysfunction of von Willebrand factor. It is not used to treat hemophilia B, which is a bleeding disorder caused by a deficiency or dysfunction of factor IX. It is not used to treat factor X or factor XI deficiencies, which are rare bleeding disorders caused by deficiencies or dysfunctions of factor X or factor XI, respectively.

SBQ 71: d) Transfusion-related acute lung injury

Transfusion-related acute lung injury (TRALI) is a rare but serious complication of blood transfusion that occurs when the donor's antibodies react with the recipient's leukocytes and cause pulmonary inflammation and edema. It is characterized by dyspnea, wheezes, hypoxia, and bilateral pulmonary infiltrates, and usually occurs within 6 hours of the transfusion. It is the leading cause of transfusion-related mortality. The treatment consists of oxygen, supportive care, and corticosteroids.

SBQ 72: d) Bacterial contamination

Bacterial contamination is a rare but serious complication of blood transfusion that occurs when the blood product contains bacteria, usually due to improper storage or handling. It is more common with platelets and plasma than with red blood cells. It is characterized by fever, chills, hypotension, and tachycardia, and usually occurs within minutes of the transfusion. It can lead to septic shock and multiorgan failure. The treatment consists of blood cultures, antibiotics, and supportive care.

SBQ 73: c) Because O negative is the universal donor for platelets

O negative is the universal donor for platelets because it does not have any ABO or Rh antigens that can cause an immune reaction in the recipient. Platelets do have ABO and Rh antigens, but they are less immunogenic than red blood cells. AB positive is the universal recipient for red blood cells, but not for platelets, because the plasma in platelets can contain anti-A and anti-B antibodies that can cause a hemolytic reaction in the recipient. The plasma volume in platelets is not negligible, and it should be compatible with the recipient's blood group.

SBQ 74: c) To detect any unexpected antibodies in the patient's plasma.

The crossmatch test is a laboratory test that is performed before a blood transfusion to ensure the compatibility of the donor's red blood cells and the recipient's plasma. It involves mixing a sample of the donor's red blood cells with a sample of the recipient's plasma and observing for any agglutination or hemolysis, which indicates an immune reaction. The crossmatch test is used to detect any unexpected antibodies in the recipient's plasma that may react with the donor's red blood cells, such as antibodies against minor blood group antigens or antibodies that develop after previous transfusions or pregnancies. The crossmatch test is not used to confirm the blood group of the donor or the recipient, as this is done by the ABO and Rh typing tests. The crossmatch test is not used to detect any hemolysis in the recipient's red blood cells, as this is done by the direct antiglobulin test.

SBQ 75: c) Plasma

Cryoprecipitate is a blood product that is derived from plasma, which is the liquid part of the blood that contains proteins, electrolytes, and clotting factors. Cryoprecipitate is obtained by freezing and thawing plasma, which causes the precipitation of a fraction that contains high concentrations of factor VIII, fibrinogen, von Willebrand factor, and factor XIII. Cryoprecipitate is used to treat bleeding disorders that involve the deficiency or dysfunction of these factors, such as hemophilia A, von Willebrand disease, and factor XIII deficiency. Cryoprecipitate is not derived from red blood cells, platelets, granulocytes, or stem cells, which are other types of blood components that have different functions and indications.

SBQ 76: b) Thalassemia

Thalassemia is a group of inherited disorders of hemoglobin synthesis that result in reduced or absent production of one or more globin chains. It is common in people of Mediterranean, African, Asian, or Middle Eastern descent. It is characterized by microcytic, hypochromic anemia with target cells and basophilic stippling on the peripheral blood smear. The serum iron, total iron-binding capacity, and ferritin levels are normal or elevated, reflecting the increased absorption of iron due to ineffective erythropoiesis. The diagnosis can be confirmed by hemoglobin electrophoresis, which shows an abnormal pattern of hemoglobin fractions.

SBQ 77: a) Acute lymphoblastic leukemia

Acute lymphoblastic leukemia (ALL) is the most common type of leukemia in children, accounting for about 80% of cases. It is caused by the clonal proliferation of immature lymphoid cells in the bone marrow and peripheral blood. It typically presents with fever, malaise, bone pain, lymphadenopathy, hepatosplenomegaly, and bleeding manifestations. The complete blood count shows pancytopenia with blasts. The peripheral blood smear shows lymphoblasts, which are large, immature cells with high nuclear-to-cytoplasmic ratio, fine chromatin, and inconspicuous nucleoli. The bone marrow biopsy shows hypercellularity with > 20% blasts. The immunophenotyping shows positive staining for CD19, CD10, CD34, and TdT, which are markers of B-cell lineage.

SBQ 78: a) Hereditary spherocytosis

Hereditary spherocytosis is a common inherited disorder of red blood cell membrane that results in the production of spherical, rather than biconcave, red blood cells. It is caused by mutations in genes encoding for membrane proteins, such as spectrin, ankyrin, or band 3. It is characterized by hemolytic anemia, jaundice, and splenomegaly. The peripheral blood smear shows spherocytes, which are small, round, and lack central pallor, polychromasia, which indicates increased reticulocytes, and Howell-Jolly bodies, which are nuclear remnants that are normally removed by the spleen. The serum bilirubin level is elevated, mainly due to indirect bilirubin, which reflects the increased breakdown of red blood cells. The serum lactate dehydrogenase level is also elevated, which reflects the increased turnover of red blood cells. The direct antiglobulin test is negative, ruling out immune-mediated hemolysis.

SBQ 79: b) Niemann-Pick disease

Niemann-Pick disease is a rare inherited disorder of lipid metabolism that results in the accumulation of sphingomyelin in various tissues, especially the liver, spleen, bone marrow, and nervous system. It is caused by mutations in genes encoding for sphingomyelinase, which is an enzyme that breaks down sphingomyelin. It is characterized by failure to thrive, hepatosplenomegaly, neurologic deterioration, and skeletal deformities. The peripheral blood smear shows normocytic, normochromic anemia with vacuolated red blood cells, and leukocytes with cytoplasmic inclusions, which are called Niemann-Pick cells. The serum acid phosphatase level is elevated, which reflects the lysosomal storage of sphingomyelin.

SBQ 80: e) Hereditary hemorrhagic telangiectasia

Hereditary hemorrhagic telangiectasia (HHT), also known as Osler-Weber-Rendu syndrome, is a rare inherited disorder of blood vessel formation that results in the development of abnormal connections between arteries and veins, called arteriovenous malformations (AVMs). It is caused by mutations in genes encoding for endoglin, activin receptor-like kinase 1, or SMAD4, which are involved in the signaling pathway of transforming growth factor beta (TGF-beta). It is characterized by recurrent epistaxis, mucocutaneous telangiectasias, and visceral AVMs, which can cause bleeding, anemia, and organ dysfunction. It can also cause short stature, due to chronic blood loss and reduced growth hormone secretion. The bleeding time is prolonged, but the coagulation tests are normal. The serum iron, total iron-binding capacity, and ferritin levels are normal, reflecting the normal synthesis and storage of iron.

SBQ 81: 1) Sickle cell anemia

Sickle cell anemia is a common inherited disorder of hemoglobin structure that results in the production of abnormal hemoglobin S, which polymerizes and deforms the red blood cells into sickle shapes under conditions of low oxygen tension. It is caused by homozygous mutations in the beta-globin gene. It is common in people of African, Mediterranean, or Middle Eastern descent. It is characterized by hemolytic anemia, jaundice, and vaso-occlusive crises, which can cause pain, organ damage, and infections. The peripheral blood smear shows normocytic, normochromic anemia with sickle cells and nucleated red blood cells, which reflect the increased erythropoiesis. The serum bilirubin level is elevated, mainly due to indirect bilirubin, which reflects the increased breakdown of red blood cells. The hemoglobin electrophoresis shows hemoglobin S of > 80% and hemoglobin F of < 20%.

SBQ 82: a) Hemophilia A

Hemophilia A is the most common inherited bleeding disorder, affecting about 1 in 5,000 male births. It is caused by a deficiency or dysfunction of factor VIII, which is a coagulation factor that participates in the intrinsic pathway of the coagulation cascade. It is characterized by deep tissue bleeding, such as hemarthrosis, muscle hematoma, and retroperitoneal bleeding, and prolonged bleeding after minor trauma or surgery. The bleeding time is normal, but the prothrombin time is normal, and the activated partial thromboplastin time is prolonged, reflecting the defect in the intrinsic pathway. The diagnosis can be confirmed by measuring the factor VIII activity level, which is low in most cases.

SBQ 83: b) Acute myeloid leukemia

Acute myeloid leukemia (AML) is a type of leukemia that occurs when the bone marrow produces abnormal myeloid cells that do not mature into normal blood cells. It is the second most common type of leukemia in children, accounting for about 20% of cases. It typically presents with fever, fatigue, bone pain, bleeding, and infection. The complete blood count shows pancytopenia with blasts. The peripheral blood smear shows myeloblasts, which are large, immature cells with high nuclear-to-cytoplasmic ratio, coarse chromatin, and prominent nucleoli. The bone marrow biopsy shows hypercellularity with > 20% blasts. The immunophenotyping shows positive staining for CD13, CD33, CD117, and MPO, which are markers of myeloid lineage.

SBQ 84: b) Thalassemia

Thalassemia is a group of inherited disorders of hemoglobin synthesis that result in reduced or absent production of one or more globin chains. It is common in people of Mediterranean, African, Asian, or Middle Eastern descent. It is characterized by microcytic, hypochromic anemia with target cells and basophilic stippling on the peripheral blood smear. The serum iron, total iron-binding capacity, and ferritin levels are normal or elevated, reflecting the increased absorption of iron due to ineffective erythropoiesis. The diagnosis can be confirmed by hemoglobin electrophoresis, which shows an abnormal pattern of hemoglobin fractions. The patient's hemoglobin electrophoresis shows hemoglobin E of 95% and hemoglobin A2 of 5%, which indicates homozygous hemoglobin E disease, a type of beta thalassemia that is common in Southeast Asia.

SBQ 85: c) Hemoglobin SC disease

Hemoglobin SC disease is a type of sickle cell disease that occurs when the patient inherits one copy of the hemoglobin S gene and one copy of the hemoglobin C gene. Hemoglobin S is an abnormal hemoglobin that polymerizes and deforms the red blood cells into sickle shapes under conditions of low oxygen tension. Hemoglobin C is an abnormal hemoglobin that crystallizes and reduces the deformability of the red blood cells. Hemoglobin SC disease is characterized by hemolytic anemia, jaundice, and vaso-occlusive crises, which can cause pain, organ damage, and infections. The peripheral blood smear shows normocytic, normochromic anemia with sickle cells and Howell-Jolly bodies, which reflect the increased erythropoiesis and the absence of the spleen. The serum bilirubin level is elevated, mainly due to indirect bilirubin, which reflects the increased breakdown of red blood cells. The hemoglobin electrophoresis shows hemoglobin S of 40-60% and hemoglobin C of 40-60%

References

1. Hoffbrand AV, Steensma DP. Hoffbrand's Essential Haematology. 8th ed. Hoboken, NJ: John Wiley & Sons Inc.; 2021.

2. Lichtman MA, Burns LJ. Initial Approach to the Patient: History and Physical Examination. In: Kaushansky K, Prchal JT, Burns LJ, Lichtman MA, Levi M, Linch DC. Eds. Williams Hematology, 10e. McGraw Hill; 2021. Accessed January 14, 2024. <https://hemonc.mhmedical.com/content.aspx?bookid=2962§ionid=252522898>

3. Carr JH, Rodak BF. Clinical Hematology Atlas. 5th ed. St. Louis, MO: Elsevier Saunders; 2020.

4. Arber DA, Orazi A, Hasserjian R, Thiele J, Borowitz MJ, Bloomfield CD, et al. The 2016 revision to the World Health Organization classification of myeloid neoplasms and acute leukemia. Blood. 2016;127(20):2391-2405. doi:10.1182/blood-2016-03-643544

5. Shander A, Cappellini MD, Goodnough LT. Iron overload and toxicity: the hidden risk of multiple blood transfusions. Vox Sanguinis. 2009;97(3):185-197. doi:10.1111/j.1423-0410.2009.01207.x

6. Khorana AA, Kuderer NM, Culakova E, Lyman GH, Francis CW. Development and validation of a predictive model for chemotherapy-associated thrombosis. Blood. 2008;111(10):4902-4907. doi:10.1182/blood-2007-10-116327

7. Narayan R, Blonquist TM, Emadi A, et al. Phase 1 study of the antibody-drug conjugate brentuximab vedotin with re-induction chemotherapy in patients with CD30-expressing relapsed/refractory acute myeloid leukemia. Cancer. 2020;126(6):1264-1273. doi:10.1002/cncr.32657

8. Palumbo A, Avet-Loiseau H, Oliva S, et al. Revised International Staging System for Multiple Myeloma: A Report From the International Myeloma Working Group. Journal of Clinical Oncology. 2015;33(26):2863-2869. doi:10.1200/JCO.2015.61.2267

9. Döhner H, Estey EH, Amadori S, et al. Diagnosis and management of acute myeloid leukemia in adults: recommendations from an international expert panel, on behalf of the European LeukemiaNet. Blood. 2010;115(3):453-474. doi:<https://doi.org/10.1182/blood-2009-07-235358>

10. Chari A, Martinez-Lopez J, Mateos MV, et al. Daratumumab Plus Carfilzomib and Dexamethasone in Patients with Relapsed or Refractory Multiple Myeloma. Blood. 2019;134(5):421-431. doi:10.1182/blood.2019000722

11. Hiddemann W, Kneba M, Dreyling M, et al. Frontline therapy with rituximab added to the combination of cyclophosphamide, doxorubicin, vincristine, and prednisone (CHOP) significantly improves the outcome for patients with advanced-stage follicular lymphoma compared with therapy with CHOP alone: results of a prospective randomized study of the German

Low-Grade Lymphoma Study Group. Blood. 2005;106(12):3725-3732. doi:10.1182/blood-2005-01-0016

12. Sasaki K, Jabbour EJ, Ravandi F, et al. Hyper-CVAD Plus Ponatinib Versus Hyper-CVAD Plus Dasatinib as Frontline Therapy for Patients with Philadelphia Chromosome-Positive Acute Lymphoblastic Leukemia: A Propensity Score Analysis. Cancer. 2016;122(23):3650-3656. doi:10.1002/cncr.30231

13. Advani RH, Moskowitz AJ, Bartlett NL, et al. Brentuximab vedotin in combination with nivolumab in relapsed or refractory Hodgkin lymphoma: 3-year study results. Blood. 2021;138(6):427-438. doi:10.1182/blood.2020009178

14. Kharfan-Dabaja MA, Kumar A, Hamadani M, et al. Clinical Practice Recommendations on Indication and Timing of Hematopoietic Cell Transplantation in Mature T Cell and NK/T Cell Lymphomas: An International Collaborative Effort on Behalf of the Guidelines Committee of the American Society for Blood and Marrow Transplantation. Biology of Blood and Marrow Transplantation. 2017;23(8):1201-1212. doi:10.1016/j.bbmt.2017.07.027

15. Lindsley RC, Saber W, Mar BG, et al. Prognostic Mutations in Myelodysplastic Syndrome after Stem-Cell Transplantation. N Engl J Med. 2017;376(6):536-547. doi:10.1056/NEJMoa1611604

16. Hoffman R, Benz EJ Jr, Silberstein LE, Heslop HE, Weitz JI, Anastasi J. Hematology: Basic Principles and Practice. 6th ed. Elsevier Saunders; 2018.

17. Kaushansky K, Lichtman MA, Prchal JT, Levi MM, Caligiuri MA, Williams ME. Williams Hematology. 10th ed. McGraw-Hill Education; 2020.

18. Sharma SK, Singh PK. Postgraduate Review Series: MCQs in Hematology. Jaypee Brothers Medical Publishers; 2021.

19. Smith AB, Johnson CD. Multiple Choice Questions for Haematology and Core Medical Trainees. 2nd ed. CRC Press; 2022.

EMQ 1

A. 2: A 67-year-old man with fatigue, pallor, and macrocytic red blood cells. His serum vitamin B12   level is low.

B. 1: A 45-year-old woman with heavy menstrual bleeding, spoon-shaped nails, and microcytic hypochromic red blood cells. Her serum ferritin level is low.

C. 4: A 32-year-old man with jaundice, splenomegaly, and spherocytic red blood cells. His direct antiglobulin test is negative.

D. 3: A 25-year-old woman with paresthesias, glossitis, and macrocytic red blood cells. Her serum folate level is low.

E. 5: A 21-year-old man with sickle cell disease, vaso-occlusive crisis, and normocytic normochromic red blood cells. His hemoglobin electrophoresis shows hemoglobin S.

EMQ 2

A. 3: A 72-year-old woman with rheumatoid arthritis, normocytic normochromic anemia, and low serum iron and transferrin levels.

B. 2: A 65-year-old man with gastric adenocarcinoma, microcytic hypochromic anemia, and low serum iron and ferritin levels.

C. 1: A 55-year-old woman with pernicious anemia, macrocytic anemia, and low serum vitamin B12 and intrinsic factor levels.

D. 4: A 35-year-old man with alcoholism, macrocytic anemia, and low serum folate and red blood cell folate levels.

E. 5: A 25-year-old woman with systemic lupus erythematosus, hemolytic anemia, and positive direct antiglobulin test.

EMQ 3

A. 2: A 22-year-old woman with thalassemia minor, microcytic hypochromic anemia, and normal serum iron and ferritin levels.

B. 1: A 18-year-old man with glucose-6-phosphate dehydrogenase deficiency, hemolytic anemia, and Heinz bodies on peripheral blood smear.

C. 4: A 27-year-old woman with iron deficiency anemia, microcytic hypochromic anemia, and low serum iron and ferritin levels.

D. 3: A 62-year-old man with myelodysplastic syndrome, macrocytic anemia, and dysplastic cells on peripheral blood smear.

E. 5: A 52-year-old woman with aplastic anemia, pancytopenia, and low reticulocyte count.

EMQ 4:

A. 1: A 42-year-old woman with iron deficiency anemia due to menorrhagia.

B. 3: A 37-year-old man with vitamin B12 deficiency anemia due to Crohn's disease.

C. 2: A 28-year-old woman with sickle cell anemia and recurrent pain crises.

D. 5: A 24-year-old man with hemolytic anemia due to warm autoimmune hemolysis.

E. 4: A 19-year-old woman with severe aplastic anemia and matched sibling donor.

EMQ 5

A. 5: A 67-year-old man with pernicious anemia and neurological symptoms.
B. 4: A 58-year-old woman with iron deficiency anemia and dysphagia.
C. 3: A 48-year-old man with hemolytic anemia and cholelithiasis.
D. 2: A 38-year-old woman with sickle cell anemia and acute chest syndrome.
E. 1: A 28-year-old man with thalassemia major and hepatomegaly.

EMQ 6:

A. 2: A 25-year-old woman with a history of systemic lupus erythematosus, who presents with fever, sore throat, and fatigue. Her WBC count is 2.1 x 10^9/L, with 60% neutrophils, 30% lymphocytes, 8% monocytes, and 2% eosinophils.
B. 3: A 35-year-old man with a history of Crohn's disease, who is on corticosteroid therapy. His WBC count is 18.5 x 10^9/L, with 80% neutrophils, 15% lymphocytes, 4% monocytes, and 1% eosinophils.
C. 1: A 45-year-old woman with a history of recurrent urinary tract infections, who presents with dysuria, frequency, and flank pain. Her WBC count is 22.3 x 10^9/L, with 88% neutrophils, 8% lymphocytes, 3% monocytes, and 1% eosinophils.
D. 4: A 55-year-old man with a history of alcoholism, who presents with macrocytic anemia and glossitis. His WBC count is 4.8 x 10^9/L, with 40% neutrophils, 50% lymphocytes, 8% monocytes, and 2% eosinophils. His neutrophils have more than five nuclear lobes.
E. 5: A 65-year-old woman with a history of rheumatoid arthritis, who is on methotrexate therapy. Her WBC count is 3.2 x 10^9/L, with 50% neutrophils, 40% lymphocytes, 8% monocytes, and 2% eosinophils. Her neutrophils have two round lobes connected by a thin filament.

EMQ7

A. 3: A 12-year-old boy with a history of asthma and allergic rhinitis, who presents with wheezing, coughing, and nasal congestion. His WBC count is 9.8 x 10^9/L, with 10% eosinophils.
B. 1: A 22-year-old woman with a history of travel to Africa, who presents with abdominal pain, diarrhea, and weight loss. Her stool examination reveals eggs of Schistosoma mansoni. Her WBC count is 11.2 x 10^9/L, with 15% eosinophils.
C. 5: A 32-year-old man with a history of ulcerative colitis, who presents with bloody stools, abdominal cramps, and fever. His WBC count is 12.5 x 10^9/L, with 12% eosinophils.
D. 4: A 42-year-old woman with a history of chronic cough, dyspnea, and skin rash. Her chest X-ray shows bilateral pulmonary infiltrates. Her WBC count is 13.4 x 10^9/L, with 18% eosinophils. Her serum IgE level is elevated.
E. 2: A 52-year-old man with a history of splenomegaly, hepatomegaly, and thrombocytopenia. His bone marrow biopsy shows increased eosinophils

and mast cells. His WBC count is 15.6 x 10^9/L, with 20% eosinophils. He has a positive test for FIP1L1-PDGFRA fusion gene.

EMQ 8

A. 1: A 16-year-old girl with a history of sore throat, fever, and malaise. Her WBC count is 14.2 x 10^9/L, with 60% lymphocytes. Her lymphocytes are large, with abundant cytoplasm and irregular nuclei.

B. 3: A 26-year-old man with a history of HIV infection, who presents with oral candidiasis, diarrhea, and weight loss. His CD4+ T cell count is 150 cells/microliter. His WBC count is 3.8 x 10^9/L, with 20% lymphocytes. His lymphocytes are small, with scanty cytoplasm and round nuclei.

C. 5: A 36-year-old woman with a history of autoimmune hemolytic anemia, who presents with fatigue, pallor, and jaundice. Her WBC count is 12.4 x 10^9/L, with 70% lymphocytes. Her lymphocytes are small to medium, with clumped chromatin and irregular nuclei. Some lymphocytes have projections or villi on their surface.

D. 4: A 46-year-old man with a history of night sweats, weight loss, and lymphadenopathy. His WBC count is 25.6 x 10^9/L, with 80% lymphocytes. His lymphocytes are small, with dense chromatin and indented nuclei. Some lymphocytes have cytoplasmic fragments or projections.

E. 2: A 56-year-old woman with a history of splenomegaly, leukocytosis, and thrombocytosis. Her WBC count is 45.2 x 10^9/L, with 40% lymphocytes. Her lymphocytes are large, with abundant cytoplasm and round or oval nuclei. Some lymphocytes have granules in their cytoplasm.

EMQ 9

A. 2: A 6-year-old boy with a history of fever, bone pain, and gingival bleeding. His WBC count is 65.4 x 10^9/L, with 40% monocytes. His monocytes are large, with folded nuclei and fine granules. His bone marrow biopsy shows increased blasts with monocytic differentiation.

B. 3: A 66-year-old man with a history of fatigue, weight loss, and splenomegaly. His WBC count is 12.8 x 10^9/L, with 15% monocytes. His monocytes are normal in size and morphology. His bone marrow biopsy shows increased monocytes and dysplasia in erythroid and megakaryocytic lineages.

C. 4: A 76-year-old woman with a history of hypertension, diabetes, and coronary artery disease, who presents with chest pain, dyspnea, and diaphoresis. Her WBC count is 14.2 x 10^9/L, with 12% monocytes. Her monocytes are normal in size and morphology. Her cardiac enzymes are elevated.

D. 1: A 86-year-old man with a history of chronic lymphocytic leukemia, who presents with fever, chills, and night sweats. His WBC count is 98.6 x 10^9/L, with 10% monocytes. His monocytes are normal in size and morphology. His blood culture is positive for Staphylococcus aureus.

E. 5: A 96-year-old woman with a history of osteoarthritis, who presents with joint pain, stiffness, and swelling. Her WBC count is 11.4 x 10^9/L, with 14%

monocytes. Her monocytes are normal in size and morphology. Her rheumatoid factor and anti-citrullinated peptide antibodies are positive

EMQ 10

A. 2: A 65-year-old man with fatigue, weight loss, and night sweats. His CBC shows leukocytosis with 90% lymphocytes, some of which have smudge cells. His flow cytometry shows CD5, CD19, and CD23 positive cells.

B. 3: A 25-year-old woman with fever, bone pain, and gingival bleeding. Her CBC shows pancytopenia with 80% blasts, some of which have Auer rods. Her cytogenetics show t(15;17).

C. 4: A 35-year-old man with pruritus, lymphadenopathy, and splenomegaly. His CBC shows normocytic anemia and eosinophilia. His biopsy shows Reed-Sternberg cells. His immunohistochemistry shows CD15 and CD30 positive cells.

D. 5: A 45-year-old woman with bone pain, renal failure, and hypercalcemia. Her CBC shows normocytic anemia and rouleaux formation. Her serum protein electrophoresis shows a monoclonal spike. Her bone marrow biopsy shows plasma cells.

E. 6: A 55-year-old man with fatigue, splenomegaly, and leukocytosis. His CBC shows increased red blood cells, white blood cells, and platelets. His JAK2 mutation test is positive.

F. 1: A 15-year-old boy with fever, lymphadenopathy, and hepatosplenomegaly. His CBC shows leukocytosis with 85% lymphoblasts. His flow cytometry shows CD10, CD19, and TdT positive cells. His cytogenetics show t(12;21).

EMQ 11

A. 4: Acute lymphoblastic leukemia (ALL).

B. 3: Chronic lymphocytic leukemia (CLL).

C. 2: Acute myeloid leukemia (AML).

D. 1: Hodgkin lymphoma.

E. 5: Multiple myeloma.

F. 6: Polycythemia vera

EMQ 12

A. 1: Acute lymphoblastic leukemia (ALL).

B. 3: Chronic lymphocytic leukemia (CLL).

C. 2: Acute myeloid leukemia (AML).

D. 6: Hodgkin lymphoma.

E. 4: Multiple myeloma.

F. 5: Mantle cell lymphoma.

EMQ 13

A. 2: Acute lymphoblastic leukemia (ALL).

B. 1: Chronic lymphocytic leukemia (CLL).

C. 4: Acute myeloid leukemia (AML).

D. 3: Hodgkin lymphoma.

E. 5: Multiple myeloma.

F. 6: Follicular lymphoma.

EMQ 14

A. 1: Acute lymphoblastic leukemia (ALL).

B. 2: Chronic lymphocytic leukemia (CLL).

C. 3: Acute myeloid leukemia (AML).

D. 4: Hodgkin lymphoma.

E. 5: Multiple myeloma.

F. 6: Polycythemia vera.

EMQ 15

A. 2: A 32-year-old woman who lives in a high-altitude area and has a history of chronic smoking. She presents with headache, dizziness, and fatigue. Her hemoglobin is 18.5 g/dL and her hematocrit is 55%. Her serum erythropoietin level is normal.

B. 2: A 42-year-old man who has a history of chronic obstructive pulmonary disease. He presents with dyspnea, cyanosis, and clubbing. His hemoglobin is 19.2 g/dL and his hematocrit is 57%. His serum erythropoietin level is elevated.

C. 1: A 52-year-old woman who has a history of hypertension and diabetes. She presents with pruritus, abdominal pain, and splenomegaly. Her hemoglobin is 20.4 g/dL and her hematocrit is 60%. Her serum erythropoietin level is low. She has a positive test for JAK2 mutation.

EMQ 16

A. 2: A 62-year-old woman who has polycythemia vera and a history of recurrent thrombosis. She presents with chest pain and shortness of breath. Her hemoglobin is 21.6 g/dL and her hematocrit is 64%. She has a positive test for JAK2 mutation.

B. 3: A 72-year-old man who has secondary polycythemia due to renal cell carcinoma. He presents with hematuria, flank pain, and weight loss. His hemoglobin is 18.8 g/dL and his hematocrit is 56%. His serum erythropoietin level is elevated.

C. 4: A 82-year-old woman who has relative polycythemia due to dehydration. She presents with confusion, dry mouth, and constipation. Her hemoglobin is 17.2 g/dL and her hematocrit is 52%. Her serum erythropoietin level is normal.

D. 5: A 92-year-old man who has polycythemia vera and a history of peptic ulcer disease. He presents with melena, anemia, and iron deficiency. His hemoglobin is 16.4 g/dL and his hematocrit is 49%. He has a positive test for JAK2 mutation.

E. 1: A 22-year-old woman who has secondary polycythemia due to congenital heart disease. She presents with cyanosis, clubbing, and palpitations. Her hemoglobin is 19.6 g/dL and her hematocrit is 58%. Her serum erythropoietin level is elevated.

EMQ 17

A. 2: A 44-year-old woman who has polycythemia vera and a history of migraine. She presents with visual disturbances, weakness, and slurred speech. Her hemoglobin is 20.8 g/dL and her hematocrit is 62%. She has a positive test for JAK2 mutation.

B. 3: A 54-year-old man who has secondary polycythemia due to sleep apnea. He presents with snoring, daytime sleepiness, and hypertension. His hemoglobin is 18.4 g/dL and his hematocrit is 55%. His serum erythropoietin level is elevated.

C. 5: A 64-year-old woman who has polycythemia vera and a history of pruritus. She presents with itching, especially after a hot shower. Her hemoglobin is 19.2 g/dL and her hematocrit is 57%. She has a positive test for JAK2 mutation.

D. 1: A 74-year-old man who has polycythemia vera and a history of gout. He presents with joint pain, swelling, and redness. His hemoglobin is 21.6 g/dL and his hematocrit is 64%. He has a positive test for JAK2 mutation.

E. 4: A 84-year-old woman who has polycythemia vera and a history of splenomegaly. She presents with abdominal discomfort, early satiety, and weight loss. Her hemoglobin is 20.4 g/dL and her hematocrit is 61%. She has a positive test for JAK2 mutation.

EMQ 18

A. 1: A 26-year-old man who has a history of living in a high-altitude area. He presents with headache, dizziness, and fatigue. His hemoglobin is 18.5 g/dL and his hematocrit is 55%. His serum erythropoietin level is normal.

B. 2: A 36-year-old woman who has a history of chronic smoking. She presents with dyspnea, cyanosis, and clubbing. Her hemoglobin is 19.2 g/dL and her hematocrit is 57%. Her serum erythropoietin level is elevated.

C. 3: A 46-year-old man who has a history of chronic obstructive pulmonary disease. He presents with cough, sputum, and wheezes. His hemoglobin is 20.4 g/dL and his hematocrit is 60%. His serum erythropoietin level is low. He has a positive test for JAK2 mutation.

D. 4: A 56-year-old woman who has a history of hypertension and diabetes. She presents with pruritus, abdominal pain, and splenomegaly. Her hemoglobin is 21.6 g/dL and her hematocrit is 64%. Her serum erythropoietin level is low. She has a positive test for JAK2 mutation.

E. 5: A 66-year-old man who has a history of renal cell carcinoma. He presents with hematuria, flank pain, and weight loss. His hemoglobin is 18.8 g/dL and his hematocrit is 56%. His serum erythropoietin level is elevated.

EMQ 19

A. 3: A 34-year-old woman who has polycythemia vera and a history of recurrent miscarriages. She presents with amenorrhea and a positive pregnancy test. Her hemoglobin is 19.6 g/dL and her hematocrit is 58%. She has a positive test for JAK2 mutation.

B. 2: A 44-year-old man who has secondary polycythemia due to sleep apnea. He presents with snoring, daytime sleepiness, and hypertension. His hemoglobin is 18.4 g/dL and his hematocrit is 55%. His serum erythropoietin level is elevated.

C. 3: A 54-year-old woman who has polycythemia vera and a history of deep vein thrombosis. She presents with leg swelling, pain, and redness. Her hemoglobin is 20.8 g/dL and her hematocrit is 62%. She has a positive test for JAK2 mutation.

D. 1: A 64-year-old man who has polycythemia vera and a history of angina. He presents with chest pain and shortness of breath. His hemoglobin is 21.6 g/dL and his hematocrit is 64%. He has a positive test for JAK2 mutation.

E. 5: A 74-year-old woman who has relative polycythemia due to dehydration. She presents with confusion, dry mouth, and constipation. Her hemoglobin is 17.2 g/dL and her hematocrit is 52%. Her serum erythropoietin level is normal.

EMQ 20:

1. B: A 25-year-old man presents with fatigue, pallor, and lymphadenopathy. Laboratory findings reveal pancytopenia, and peripheral blood film displays lymphoblasts. Immunophenotyping confirms the presence of T-cell lymphoblasts expressing CD3, CD4, and CD8.

2. C: A 60-year-old woman is diagnosed with leukemia following complaints of fatigue, bruising, and weight loss. Peripheral blood film demonstrates myeloblasts without maturation beyond the myeloblast stage. Cytogenetic analysis reveals inv(16)(p13.1q22) or t(16;16)(p13.1;q22).

3. E: A 45-year-old man is found to have leukopenia, anemia, and thrombocytopenia. Blood film reveals myeloid blasts expressing CD13, CD33, and CD117. Complex karyotype alterations are identified.

4. F: A 30-year-old woman is diagnosed with acute leukemia displaying promyelocytes with abundant azurophilic granules and Auer rods on blood film. Cytogenetic analysis reveals t(15;17)(q22;q12).

5. G: A 55-year-old man presents with extensive cutaneous involvement, marked by violaceous patches and nodules. Biopsy reveals a monomorphic infiltrate composed of medium-sized blast cells with round nuclei, finely dispersed chromatin, and indistinct nucleoli. Immunostain highlights positivity for CD4, CD56, and CD123.

EMQ 21

1. F: A 20-year-old female with Burkitt leukemia

2. B: A 50-year-old male with AML harboring FLT3 internal tandem duplication

3. E: A 30-year-old female with newly diagnosed APL

4. A: A 65-year-old male with newly diagnosed DLBCL involving bone marrow

5. D: A 40-year-old female with Ph-negative ALL having good risk characteristics.

EMQ 22
1. B: Preventing infectious complications in neutropenic patients
2. E: Managing life-threatening bleeding in a patient with profound thrombocytopenia
3. D: Addressing severe anemia in a patient with acute leukemia
4. C: Removing excess white blood cells to decrease the risk of tumor lysis syndrome
5. G: Encouraging adequate nutrition intake and preventing cachexia in patients undergoing treatment.
EMQ 23
1. A: Development of a painful, tender, warm, erythematous patch with surrounding edema in a patient with AML treated with ATRA
2. C: Sudden onset of severe headache, altered mental status, visual disturbances, and seizures in a patient with acute leukemia
3. E: Rapid reduction in urinary output, hyperkalemia, hyperphosphatemia, and hypocalcemia in a patient with acute leukemia initiating intensive chemotherapy
4. F: Progressive shortness of breath, stridor, and facial plethora in a patient with acute leukemia
5. B: New-onset pericardial friction rub, jugular venous distention, and Beck's triad in a patient with acute leukemia
EMQ 24
1. F: Craniospinal radiotherapy in a 10-year-old child with medulloblastoma
2. E: Total body irradiation prior to autologous stem cell transplantation
3. A: Maintenance chemotherapy consisting of mercaptopurine and methotrexate for a patient with ALL
4. D: High cumulative doses of anthracyclines in a patient with AML
5. C: Busulfan and cyclophosphamide conditioning regimen before allogeneic stem cell transplantation
EMQ 25
1. B: Predominantly affects elderly individuals
2. A: Presents with massive splenomegaly
3. C: Often accompanied by peripheral lymphadenopathy
4. F: Associated with skin lesions and pruritis
5. D: Can arise from hair follicles
6. A: Typically manifests as a progressive increase in absolute neutrophil count
7. B: Occurs predominately in middle-aged to older adults
EMQ 26
1. A: Constitutively active tyrosine kinase resulting in uncontrolled proliferation
2. B: Overexpression of cyclin D1 promoting entry into the cell cycle
3. C: Formation of MYC-IGH fusion protein driving lymphocyte transformation

4. F: Mutation commonly observed in CLL/SLL, particularly in familial cases

5. E: Aberrant expression of runt-related transcription factor 1

6. D: Triplicated allele seen in approximately 15–20% of CLL cases

7. G: Somatic mutation occurring in around half of CLL/SLL patients

EMQ 27

1. B: Detecting submicroscopic deletions in del(17p) or del(11q)

2. A: Identifying reciprocal translocation between chromosomes 9 and 22

3. F: Quantitating BCR: ABL1 transcripts

4. D: Assessing the clonal expansion of lymphocytes

5. F: Screening for the presence of the Philadelphia chromosome

6. C: Determining the somatic mutations present in leukemic cells

EMQ 28

1. F: Frontline management for asymptomatic, stable-phase CML

2. D: Treatment for newly diagnosed mantle cell lymphoma

3. F: Initial therapy for previously untreated CLL/SLL

4. E: Optimal treatment for young, fit patients with advanced-stage FL

5. C: Standard of care for CD52-positive CLL/SLL

EMQ 29

1. A: Treatment for CML refractory to imatinib

2. D: Treatment for CLL/SLL with del(17p)

3. C: Monotherapy for CLL/SLL carrying TP53 or SF3B1 mutations

4. B: Targeted agent approved for both CLL/SLL and mantle cell lymphoma

5. G: Agent combined with rituximab for treating FL

1. A: A 60-year-old male lifelong smoker presenting with plethoric facies and erythrocytosis

2. B: A 45-year-old obese male experiencing sleep apnea and concomitant erythrocytosis

3. G: A 35-year-old resident living near sea level complaining of fatigue, dyspnea, and erythrocytosis

4. D: A 50-year-old female suffering from renovascular hypertension caused by renal artery stenosis and accompanying erythrocytosis

5. E: A 70-year-old male taking testosterone replacement therapy and developing erythrocytosis

EMQ 31

1. C: A 65-year-old male with weakness, dyspnea, and dark urine

2. B: A 70-year-old female suffering from sudden bone pain and collapse

3. F: A 55-year-old male with recurrent upper respiratory tract infections

4. G: A 60-year-old female with decreasing estimated glomerular filtration rate (eGFR)

5. E: A 75-year-old male with spontaneous bleeds and petechiae

EMQ 32

1. B: A 60-year-old male with albumin 4.5 g/dL, beta-2 microglobulin 2.5 mg/L, and normal lactic dehydrogenase (LDH)

2. A: A 55-year-old female with albumin 3.2 g/dL, beta-2 microglobulin 4.0 mg/L, and normal LDH

3. C: A 65-year-old male with albumin 2.8 g/dL, beta-2 microglobulin 6.0 mg/L, and elevated LDH

EMQ 33

1. B: A 60-year-old otherwise healthy female seeking aggressive treatment

2. A: An 80-year-old male with significant comorbidities and limited functional ability

3. C: A 75-year-old male with slow-progressing multiple myeloma

EMQ 34

1. A: Destruction of bone matrix releasing calcium

2. E: Accumulation of light chains in the tubular lumina

3. G: Impairment of humoral and cell-mediated immunity

4. D: Suppression of erythropoiesis due to bone marrow invasion

5. E: Elevation of Bence Jones protein hindering renal clearance

6. F: Crowded vessels reducing blood flow velocity

7. B: Production of ammonia by urea-splitting bacteria

EMQ 35

1. A: Reed-Sternberg cells

2. C: Germinal centers containing centroblasts and centrocytes

3. D: Most common primary extranodal site being the ocular adnexae

4. E: Usually low grade with an indolent course

5. F: Associated with the characteristic t(11;14)(q13;q32) translocation

EMQ 36

1. B: Two or more lymph node regions on the same side of the diaphragm involved

2. A: Single lymph node region or single extra-nodal organ affected

3. D: Diffuse involvement of one or more organs outside the lymphatic system

4. C: Lymph node regions on both sides of the diaphragm involved

EMQ 37

1. C: B-cell lymphomas

2. D: T-cell lymphomas

3. F: Hodgkin lymphoma

4. E: Anaplastic large cell lymphoma

5. G: Multiple myeloma

EMQ 38

1. A: Mantle cell lymphoma is characterized by the t(11;14) translocation that results in overexpression of CCND1, a gene that encodes cyclin D1, a cell cycle regulator.

2. B: Diffuse large B-cell lymphoma is a heterogeneous group of lymphomas that often harbor mutations in TP53, a gene that encodes p53, a tumor suppressor protein. TP53 mutations are associated with poor prognosis and resistance to chemotherapy.

3. D: Follicular lymphoma is the most common indolent lymphoma that frequently involves the t(14;18) translocation that leads to overexpression of BCL2, a gene that encodes Bcl-2, an anti-apoptotic protein. BCL2 mutations confer survival advantage to the lymphoma cells.

4. E: Burkitt lymphoma is a highly aggressive lymphoma that is associated with translocations involving the MYC gene, which encodes a transcription factor that promotes cell growth and proliferation. The most common translocation partner is the BCL6 gene, which encodes a B-cell specific transcriptional repressor. BCL6 mutations are involved in the pathogenesis and progression of Burkitt lymphoma.

5. C: Waldenström macroglobulinemia is a rare type of lymphoplasmacytic lymphoma that produces excessive amounts of IgM, a type of antibody. The majority of Waldenström macroglobulinemia cases have a mutation in the MYD88 gene, which encodes a protein that mediates signaling from the B-cell receptor and Toll-like receptors. MYD88 mutations activate the NF-κB pathway and enhance the survival and growth of the lymphoma cells.

EMQ 39

1. E: Qualitative platelet disorder with decreased surface integrin αIIbβ3

2. D: Disorder characterized by giant platelets and impaired platelet aggregation

3. A: Platelets exhibit reduced dense granule release and diminished platelet activation

4. C: Congenital absence of von Willebrand factor leads to impaired platelet adhesion

5. E: Surface integrin αIIbβ3 is completely missing, resulting in severe bleeding tendencies

6. F: Platelets possess reduced amounts of dense and alpha granules

EMQ 40

1. E: Testing platelet aggregation patterns in response to specific agents

2. B: Visualizing ultrastructure of platelets to identify structural anomalies

3. D: Monitoring global clot formation dynamics in vitro

4. C: Enumerating platelet surface markers to assess platelet functionality

5. A: Estimating susceptibility to bleeding by evaluating capillary perfusion

EMQ 41

1. A: Afibrinogenemia

2. B: Type 1 von Willebrand disease

3. G: Menorrhagia induced by platelet function disorder

4. E: Severe bleeding episode in a patient with Glanzmann thrombasthenia

5. F: Preoperative preparation for a patient with platelet storage pool deficiency

EMQ 42

1. A: Coagulation disorder with a deficiency in factor VIII

2. B: Condition with reduced factor IX levels

3. D: Insufficient production of functional coagulation factors due to impaired liver synthetic capability

4. C: Syndrome caused by insufficient vitamin K availability

5. E: Inhibition of vitamin K-dependent coagulation factors due to warfarin ingestion

6. G: Diminished or dysfunctional fibrinogen molecules

7. F: Deficiency of contact phase coagulation protein

EMQ 43

1. F: Assessment of factor VIII activity

2. B: Analysis of contact phase coagulation proteins

3. C: Global screening test for intrinsic and final common pathways

4. D: Overall measurement of the conversion of fibrinogen to fibrin

5. G: Evaluation of overall hemostatic capability including platelets and the extrinsic and common pathways

6. F: Investigation of specific factor activities

EMQ 44

1. B: Moderate to severe factor VIII deficiency

2. B: Factor IX deficiency

3. A: Mild to moderate factor deficiency with planned invasive procedure

4. D: Disseminated intravascular coagulation (DIC)

5. C: Excessive anticoagulation due to oral anticoagulant therapy

6. F: Heparin-induced thrombocytopenia (HIT)

EMQ 45

1. B: Restoration of intravascular volume

2. B: Correction of hypovolemic shock

3. A: Compensation for severe anemia

4. C: Providing clotting factors

5. D: Administering platelets

6. E: Augmenting fibrinogen levels

7. F: Infusing colloids for maintaining oncotic pressure

EMQ 46

1. A: Required for tracking purposes during recall events

2. A: Helps prevent clerical errors

3. F: Facilitates determination of remaining shelf life

4. D: Crucial for ensuring compatibility during transfusion

5. E: Important for providing type-specific products to Rh-negative females

6. C: Critical in selecting appropriate units for specific patients

7. G: Useful for efficient allocation and retrieval of blood products

EMQ 47

1. A: Before issuing blood to a new patient with unknown antibody screen results

2. B: Prior to transfusing a repeat patient whose last antibody screen showed no clinically significant antibodies

3. E: When immediate transfusion is necessary, and the automated crossmatch is delayed or unavailable

4. C: In urgent situations where rapid antibody detection is crucial

5. D: Utilizing electronic data systems for routine, elective procedures

EMQ 48

1. F: Delayed recovery from illness or operation

2. E: Respiratory distress and fluid accumulation

3. C: Acute renal failure

4. B: Shortened survival of transfused red blood cells

5. D: Life-threatening cardiopulmonary compromise

6. G: Bronchospasm, hives, or angioedema

7. A: Possibility of acquiring fatal or debilitating infections

EMQ 49

1. A: Red blood cell substitute

2. C: Fibrin sealant

3. D: Apheresis-derived platelets processed to reduce bacterial burden

4. E: Devices collecting shed blood during surgical procedures for later infusion

5. B: Alternative to traditional plasma derivatives

6. F: Endogenous stimulator of erythropoiesis

7. G: White blood cell removal technology

EMQ 50

1. A: Trauma patients requiring resuscitation with balanced ratios

2. B: Cardiovascular surgeries necessitating high-volume support

3. C: Orthopedic operations demanding substantial input

4. E: Jehovah's Witnesses rejecting transfusion yet needing surgical intervention

5. G: Pediatric patients undergoing extensive procedures

References

1. Rowley JD. Letter: A New Consistent Chromosomal Abnormality in Chronic Myelogenous Leukemia Identified by Quinacrine Fluorescence and Giemsa Staining. Nature. 1973;243(5405):290-293. doi:10.1038/243290a0

2. Tallman MS, Wang ES, Altman JK, et al. NCCN Clinical Practice Guidelines in Oncology: Acute Myeloid Leukemia, version 3.2019. J Natl Compr Canc Netw. 2019;17(6):721-749. doi:10.6004/jnccn.2019.0028

3. Druker BJ, Lydon NB. Lessons Learned From the Development of an ABL Tyrosine Kinase Inhibitor for Chronic Myelogenous Leukemia. J Clin Invest. 2000;105(1):3-7. doi:10.1172/JCI9083

4. Arber DA, Orazi A, Hasserjian R, et al. The 2016 Revision to the World Health Organization Classification of Myeloid Neoplasms and Acute Leukemia. Blood. 2016;127(20):2391-2405. doi:10.1182/blood-2016-03-643544

5. Montesinos P, Bergua JM, Vellenga E, et al. Differentiation Syndrome in Patients with Acute Promyelocytic Leukemia Treated with All-Trans Retinoic Acid and Anthracycline Chemotherapy: Characteristics, Outcome, and Prognostic Factors. Blood. 2009;113(4):775-783. doi:10.1182/blood-2008-07-168617

6. Cho SY, Kim SY, Jeon YL, et al. A Novel Three-Way Ph Variant t(8;9;22) in Adult Acute Lymphoblastic Leukemia. Ann Clin Lab Sci. 2011;41(1):71-78.

7. Kaleem Z, Crawford E, Pathan MH, et al. Flow Cytometric Analysis of Acute Leukemias: Diagnostic Utility and Critical Analysis of Data. Arch Pathol Lab Med. 2003;127(1):42-48. doi:10.5858/2003-127-42-FCAOA

8. Yalniz FF, Patel KP, Bashir Q, et al. Minimal Residual Disease Monitoring by Real-Time Quantitative Polymerase Chain Reaction in Core Binding Factor Acute Myeloid Leukemia for Transplantation Outcomes. Cancer. 2020;126(10):2183-2192. doi:10.1002/cncr.32769

9. Müller BJ, Inaba H. Chimeric Antigen Receptor T-Cells in B-Acute Lymphoblastic Leukemia: History, Current Situation, and Future. Transl Pediatr. 2023;12(10):1900-1907. doi:10.21037/tp-23-366

10. Barbui T, Falanga A. Disseminated Intravascular Coagulation in Acute Leukemia. Semin Thromb Hemost. 2001;27(6):593-604. doi:10.1055/s-2001-18865

11. Bakr M, Rasheed W, Mohamed SY, et al. Allogeneic Hematopoietic Stem Cell Transplantation in Adolescent and Adult Patients with High-Risk T Cell Acute Lymphoblastic Leukemia. Biol Blood Marrow Transplant. 2012;18(12):1897-1904. doi:10.1016/j.bbmt.2012.07.011

12. Levavi H, Hoffman R, Marcellino BK. Jak Inhibitors in the Treatment of Myelofibrosis. Clin Adv Hematol Oncol. 2022;20(7):456-467

13. Greenburg AG, Greer JP, Walter MH, Beutler E, Branch DJ, Faust JS. Wintrobe's Clinical Hematology. 13th ed. Wolters Kluwer; 2018.

14. Wallach J. Interpretation of Diagnostic Tests. 9th ed. Lippincott Williams & Wilkins; 2017.